A CARERS GUIDE TO YOUR OWN MENTAL HEALTH & WHAT TO EXPECT IN CARE

ME, MYSELF & THE OTHER ONE

BY ROY LANGSTAFFE

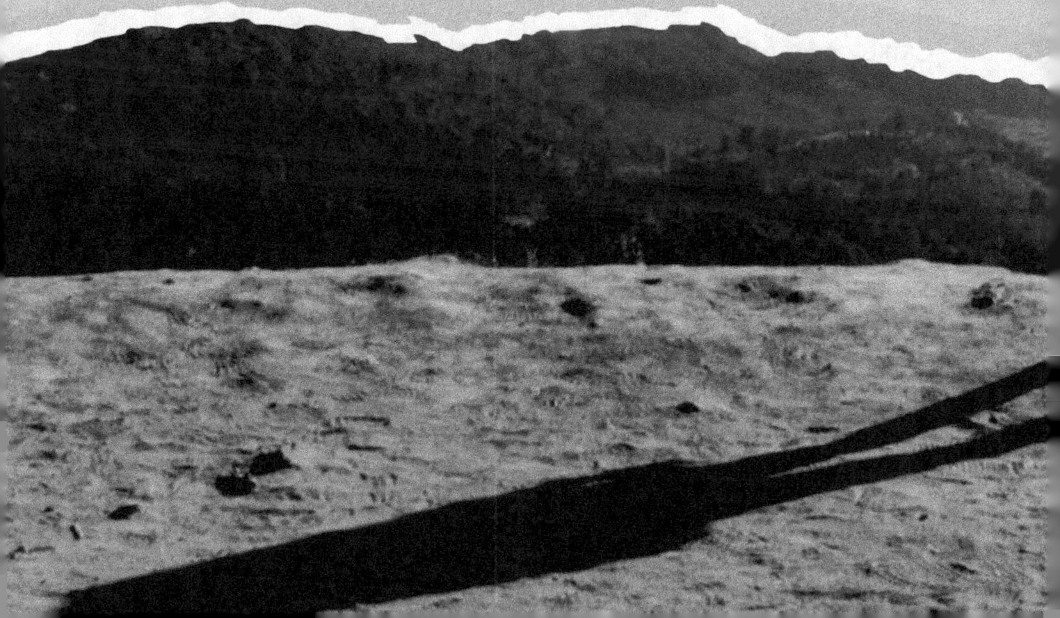

This book is dedicated to all those amazing carers out there that really make a difference. Without you THE OTHER ONE's would not have that quality of support!

ME, MYSELF & THE OTHER ONE:

A CARERS GUIDE TO MENTAL HEALTH & WHAT TO EXPECT IN CARE

Hello, I'm Roy Langstaffe, a seasoned trainer and coach with a deep passion for caregiving. With years of experience, I excel in guiding individuals to become exceptional caregivers.

I collaborate with diverse organizations to elevate caregiving standards and practices. Beyond my training endeavors, I'm also an author and aspiring musician, showcasing my multifaceted approach to life.

My commitment to the well-being of caregivers is evident in my tireless advocacy and dedication. With compassion and creativity at the forefront, I strive to make a meaningful impact on the lives of caregivers and those they care for, ensuring their sanity and strength are upheld.

I hope you enjoy this book and find some knowledge that helps you!

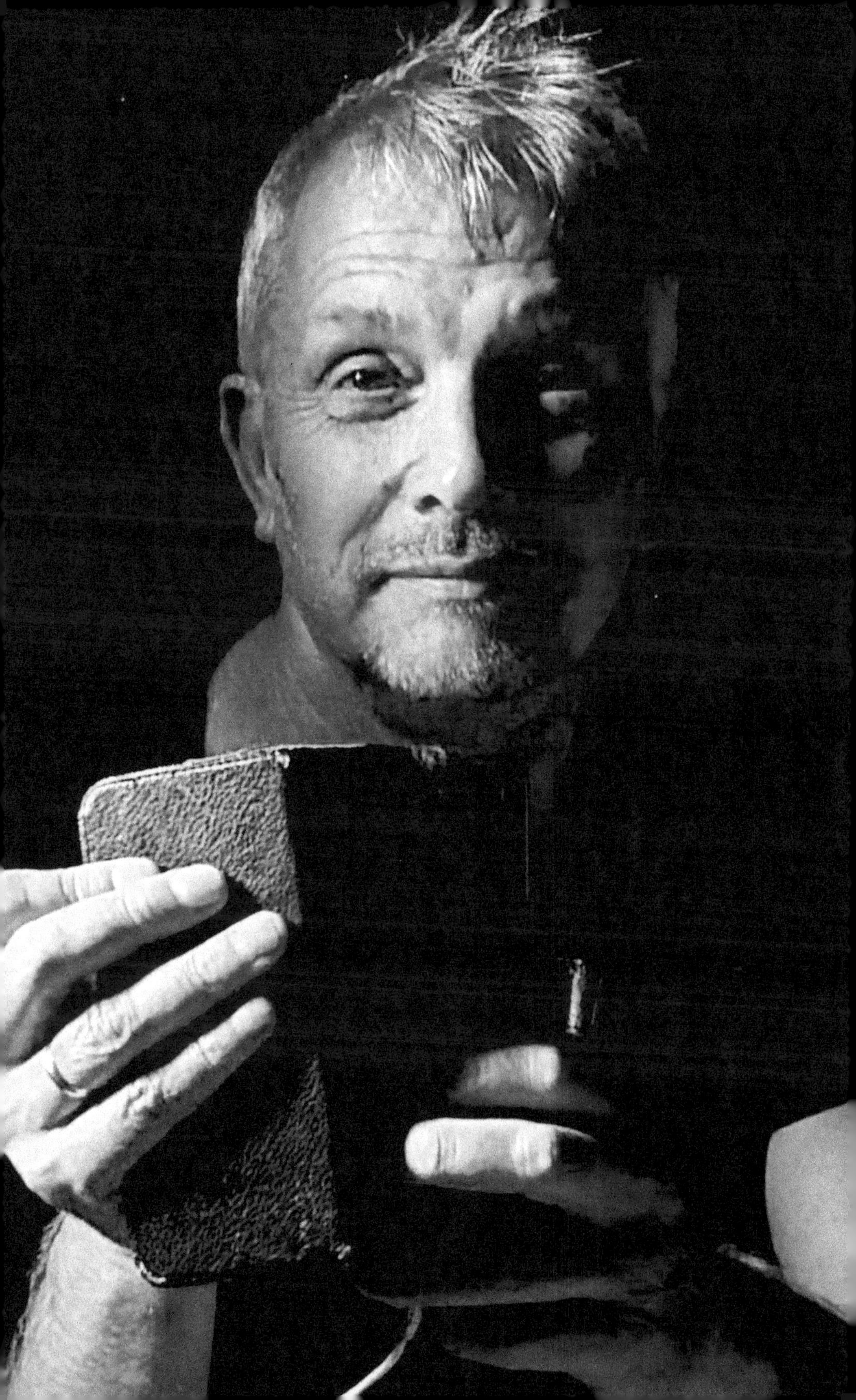

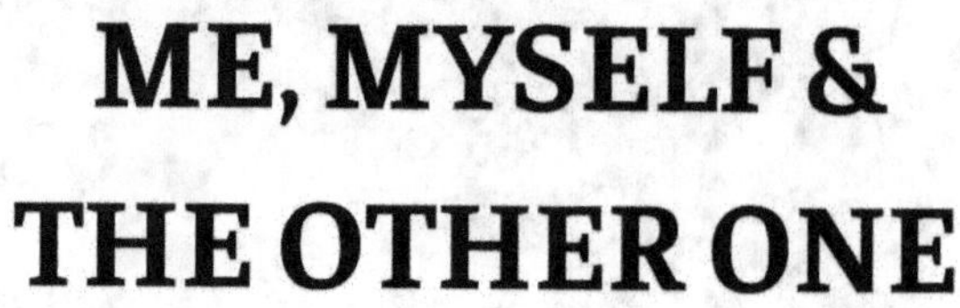

ME, MYSELF & THE OTHER ONE

A CARERS GUIDE TO YOUR OWN MENTAL HEALTH & WHAT TO EXPECT IN CARE

CONTENTS

Introduction

Chapter 1
In the Beginning

Chapter 2
Understanding Mental Health in Care Giving

Chapter 3
Do I Really Have to Do That!

Chapter 4
Stress and how it affects MYSELF

Chapter 5
Understanding Anxiety and Depression.

Chapter 6
*Building Resilience and
Emotional Well-being*

Chapter 7
*Practical Self-Care
Strategies for Caregivers*

Chapter 8
*Effective Communication
and Relationships*

Chapter 9
*Professional Help
& Resources*

Chapter 10
*Addressing Mental Health
Needs in THE OTHER ONE*

Chapter 11
Legal & Financial Considerations

Chapter 12
Long Term Care Planning

Conclusion
You, Me and THE OTHER ONE

Appendix
Acknowledgements

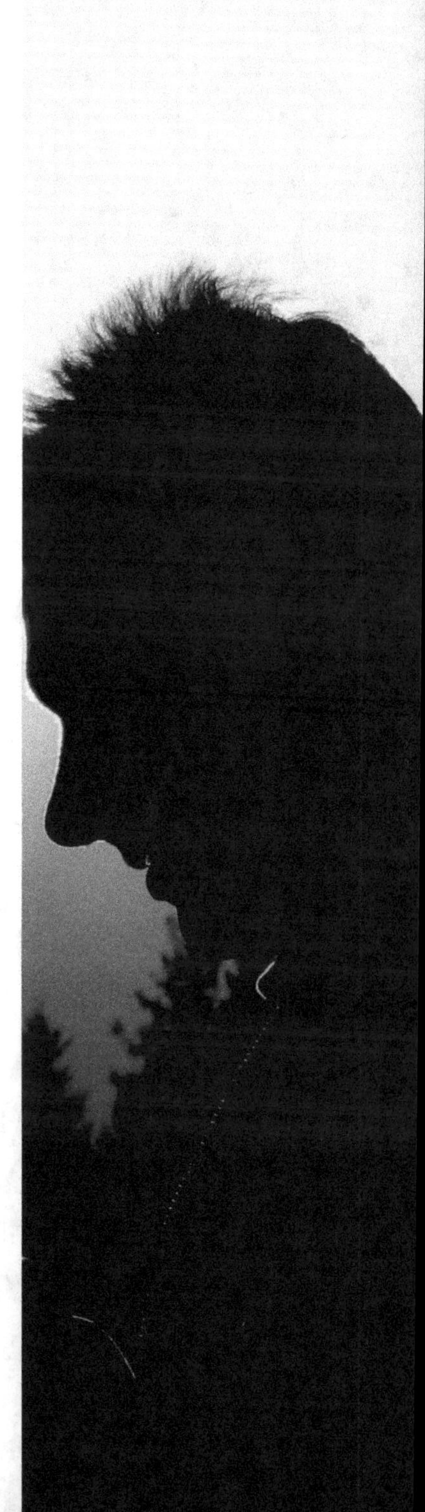

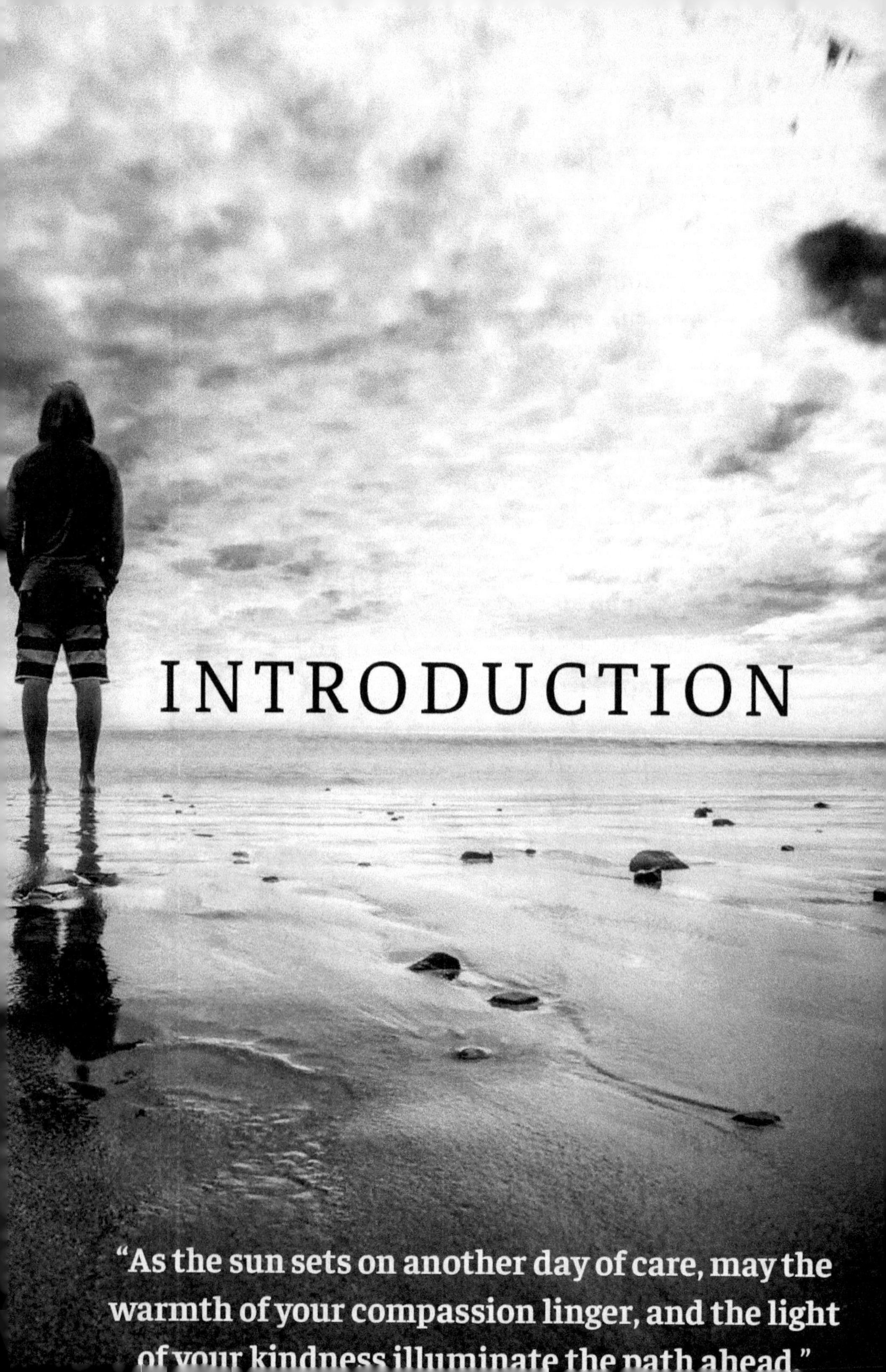

INTRODUCTION

Welcome to "Me, Myself, and the Other One: A Carer's Guide to Mental Health and What to Expect in Care."

As a seasoned caregiver with over three decades of experience, I've walked alongside countless individuals, sharing in their triumphs and challenges. Through these journeys, I've gained invaluable insights into the profound impact of caregiving on mental health—both for the caregiver and the one receiving care.

In this guide, I draw not only from my own experiences but also from the stories of those I've trained and supported. Together, we'll navigate the complexities of caregiving, shining a light on the often-overlooked aspect of mental well-being. Along the way, I'll weave in inspirational writings, quotes, and poems to uplift and guide you through this transformative journey.

Picture this: You're a caregiver, orchestrating the intricacies of daily life while providing unwavering support to a loved one. Your days blur into a whirlwind of tasks, appointments, and responsibilities. Yet, amidst this chaos, the crucial element of mental health often slips through the cracks—for both you and the person you care for.

Caregiving is undeniably rewarding, but it can also push you to your limits. The relentless demands, the emotional weight of witnessing a loved one's struggles, and the sheer exhaustion can leave you feeling adrift and overwhelmed. But why does mental health support matter so much in caregiving?

Together, we'll delve into the vital importance of prioritizing mental well-being for both caregivers and care recipients. This eBook serves as your lifeline, offering guidance as you navigate the intricate terrain of caregiving's mental health challenges.

OLI THE OCTOPUS

In the depths of the ocean, where stories unfold,
Lived Oli the Octopus, with arms brave and bold.
A multitasking carer, his duties vast,
But sometimes, oh dear, he got tangled up fast.

With eight arms a-whirling, he'd care for them all,
From fishes to crabs, he answered each call.
But in his flurry, he'd trip and he'd sway,
In a tangle of tasks, he'd lose his own way.

Yet still, he persisted, with love in his heart,
For those in his care, he'd do his part.
Though sometimes ensnared in a web of his own,
He'd free himself, determined, his spirit unblown.

So here's to Oli the Octopus, though tangled he'd be,
In caring for others, he found his decree.
A lesson for us, in the whirl of our days,
To untangle our tasks, in compassionate ways.

CHAPTER ONE

IN THE
BEGINNING

"No matter how challenging the path may be, finding moments of joy and humor can lighten the load"

1.1
So You Just Found Out

A True Story
I was told this story about someone I used to support about the day things changed for him by his friend Mark. It was a chilly autumn evening, and the leaves had just begun to fall. Simon, father of two, was found collapsed outside his home after a night at a bar. He was only 43. It was an ordinary evening turned extraordinary by an unexpected event that would forever change his life and his close friend Mark forever. The doctors later revealed that Simon had Huntington's Disease, a degenerative neurological condition. His friend explained, whom he had known all his life, as he sat by his hospital bed, a whirlwind of emotions engulfed him – fear, confusion, sadness, and oddly enough, a sense of relief. It was a defining moment, one that many people face when they first learn their friends or loved one needs care.

A Rollercoaster of Emotions
When you first find out that someone you love needs care, it's natural to feel a range of emotions. Whether it's due to an accident, a sudden diagnosis, or a gradual realization, the initial shock can be overwhelming. You might feel scared about the future, unsure about your ability to provide the care needed. At the same time, there can be a sense of relief – finally, you have answers to those unexplained symptoms or behaviours.

Fear and Uncertainty
Fear is often the first emotion that surfaces. The uncertainty of what lies ahead can be daunting. You might worry about the practical aspects – medical bills, daily routines, and long-term care plans. The thought of taking on such a significant responsibility can be terrifying. It's okay to feel scared. It's a natural reaction to stepping into the unknown. What will I (ME) have to do, how will it affect MYSELF and my mental health. How will is affect the person I will be supporting, THE OTHER ONE.

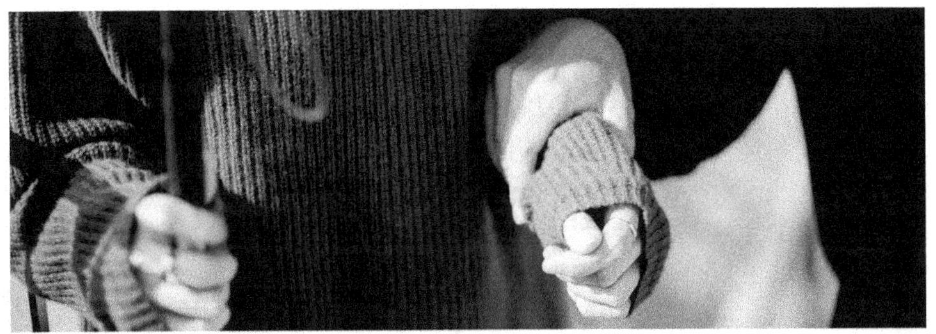

The toll of caregiving is often hidden beneath layers of responsibility and duty. Did you know that nearly one-third of caregivers report high levels of emotional stress? This stress can stem from various sources—the ceaseless nature of caregiving tasks, financial strains, and the emotional weight of witnessing a loved one's struggles.

But the repercussions of neglecting mental health can be severe. Studies reveal that caregivers experiencing chronic stress have a 23% higher level of stress hormones, predisposing them to serious health issues like heart disease and depression. These statistics underscore the urgent need for mental health support—a fundamental component of the caregiving journey.

While caregivers rightfully receive attention, it's equally crucial to consider the mental well-being of those receiving care. Chronic illness, disability, or aging can take a significant toll, leading to feelings of helplessness, isolation, and anxiety. Addressing these mental health needs isn't just compassionate—it's essential for better health outcomes and an improved quality of life.

Despite the clear need, mental health support for caregivers and care recipients often falls short. Why? Numerous barriers contribute to this gap, including stigma, lack of resources, and limited awareness. Breaking down these barriers is essential—through open dialogue, improved access to services, and education, we can bridge the mental health gap in caregiving.

Relief and Understanding

Simultaneously, you might feel a wave of relief. After months or even years of confusion, you finally have a name for what's been happening. For those dealing with conditions like Autism or Dementia, a diagnosis can provide a framework for understanding the behaviours and symptoms you've been witnessing. Simon's diagnosis of Huntington's Disease, while devastating, also brought clarity. We could now understand his erratic behaviour and physical symptoms, and they could begin to plan for the future.

Sadness and Grief

Sadness and grief are also common. You grieve for the life you thought you had, the plans you made, and the future that now looks different. It's important to allow yourself to feel this sadness. Bottling up emotions can lead to burnout and mental health issues down the line. It's okay to mourn the change and to acknowledge the loss of what once was.

Acceptance and Resolve

Over time, these emotions can lead to acceptance and resolve. Accepting the new reality doesn't mean you have to like it or agree with it, but it allows you to move forward with a sense of purpose. You begin to find strength within yourself, and a determination to provide the best care possible for your loved one.

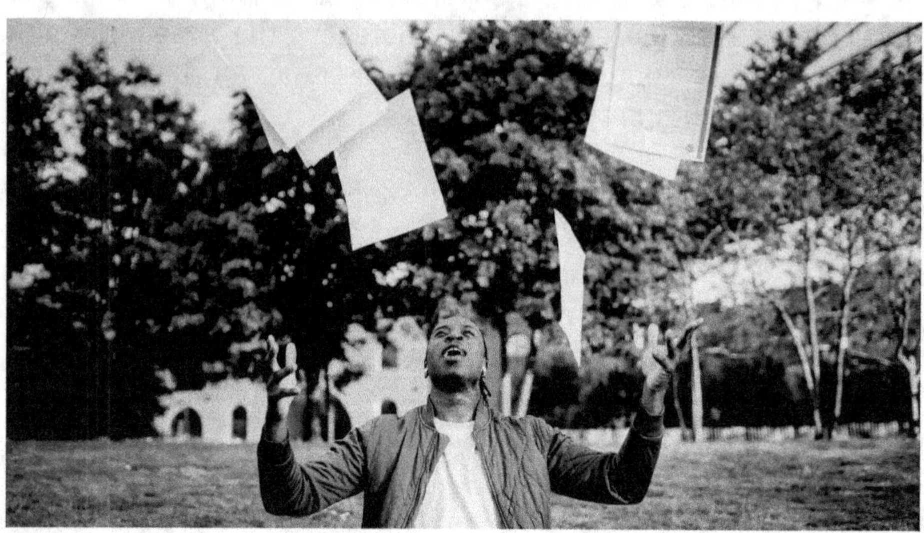

Embrace the Journey

In conclusion, finding out that your loved one needs care can be both a scary and a relieving experience. It's a journey filled with a range of emotions, from fear and sadness to relief and acceptance. Remember that it's okay to feel all these emotions and that you're not alone. By taking practical steps and building a support network, you can navigate this journey with strength and resilience. While the journey is hard, don't give up. Your perseverance makes a positive impact on both your life and your loved one's life.

Embrace each day with courage and compassion, and remember that every small victory is a step forward on this path. ME, MYSELF, and, of course, the person you are supporting, THE OTHER ONE, are really important. Celebrate the progress you make together, no matter how small, and let these moments of connection and triumph fuel your dedication.

In the face of challenges, find the strength to keep going, knowing that your unwavering support and love make a world of difference.

Start each day with "I can," not "I can't." Always say "I will," not "I won't."

As you journey through this experience, you will change, but th will be a change for the better. Your journey, though demanding, is a testament to your incredible resilience and boundless compassion, leading you to grow stronger and more compassionate every day.

Simon's Story

Let me take you back to Simon's story.

After the initial shock of his diagnosis, his family and friends went through a whirlwind of emotions. His best friend Mark was particularly affected, feeling an immense sense of responsibility to care for Simon while also being terrified of the unknown. Adding to the stress, Simon's wife, who was deeply upset, felt she could not cope and left Simon to handle the situation alone. Simon and his wife decided they didn't want their children to witness his decline, preferring they remember him as he was.

Mark's journey, like that of many caregivers, began with fear but gradually shifted towards acceptance and resolve. He found strength in friendship and commitment, which made him and everyone around him stronger. Support from caregiver groups, advice from professionals, and the establishment of a routine that worked for both him and Simon became vital.

Mark learned to celebrate small victories and find joy in the moments they shared. His story is a testament to the resilience and strength caregivers can discover within themselves. Even when Simon had to enter a care facility, Mark's commitment never wavered. He visited every Friday for a beer and to remind Simon that he was never alone.

This story illustrates how friendship and commitment can fortify us, making us all stronger in the face of adversity. The unwavering support from friends can provide emotional stability, encouragement, and a sense of belonging, transforming difficult times into opportunities for deeper connections and shared resilience.

Due to his Huntington's Disease, Simon lost the ability to speak. In fact, the last word he ever spoke was the word BEER, probabally because his friend Mark was there for him and every Friday he always took him out for a beer.

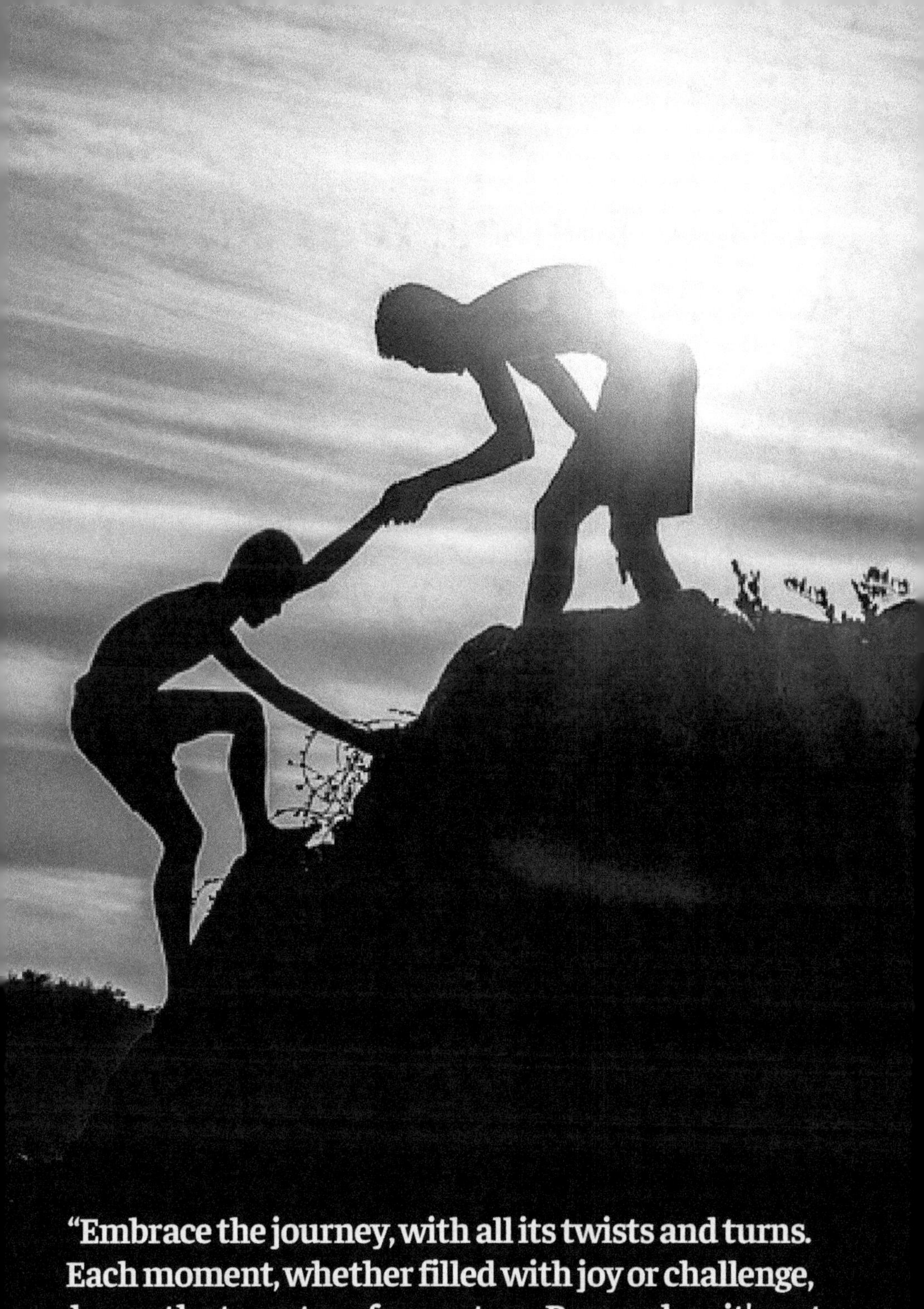

"Embrace the journey, with all its twists and turns.
Each moment, whether filled with joy or challenge,
shapes the tapestry of your story. Remember, it's not
just the destination that matters, but the strength
and friendship you discover along the way."

1.2
Prepare Yourself. You Could Be in for a Ride!

Embarking on the journey of caregiving is like setting off on an uncharted adventure. There will be moments of joy and deep connection, but there will also be challenges and unexpected turns. The key to navigating this journey successfully lies in preparation and maintaining a calm and steady approach. As you step into this role, it's crucial to arm yourself with knowledge, build a support network, and stay mentally and emotionally resilient. In this module, we'll discuss how to prepare yourself for the caregiving journey ahead.

Understanding the Importance of Preparation

Preparation is the foundation upon which successful caregiving is built. It allows you to anticipate challenges, manage stress, and provide the best possible care for your loved one. By taking the time to prepare, you can approach caregiving with confidence and a sense of control, rather than feeling overwhelmed and reactive.

ME: What Do I Need to Prepare?

Gathering Information

Learn About the Condition: Educate yourself about the specific condition your loved one is facing. Whether it's Autism, Dementia, Huntington's Disease, or another condition, understanding the symptoms, progression, and treatment options is crucial. This knowledge will help you make informed decisions and provide appropriate care.

Stay Informed: Keep up to date with the latest research, treatments, and caregiving strategies. Join online forums, subscribe to newsletters, and participate in webinars to stay informed.

ME: What Does This All Mean to Me?

Understanding the condition is just the beginning. Reflect on how this new role will impact your daily life, your emotions, and your mental health. Ask yourself:

- How will my daily routine change?
- What new skills do I need to learn?
- How will this affect my work and social life?

Building a Support Network

One of the key things to do is to build a support network. ME will need it!

Family and Friends: Engage family members and friends in the caregiving process. Share responsibilities and communicate openly about the challenges you're facing. A strong support network can provide emotional support and practical assistance.

Support Groups: Join caregiver support groups, either in person or online. Connecting with others who are in similar situations can provide invaluable advice, empathy, and encouragement.

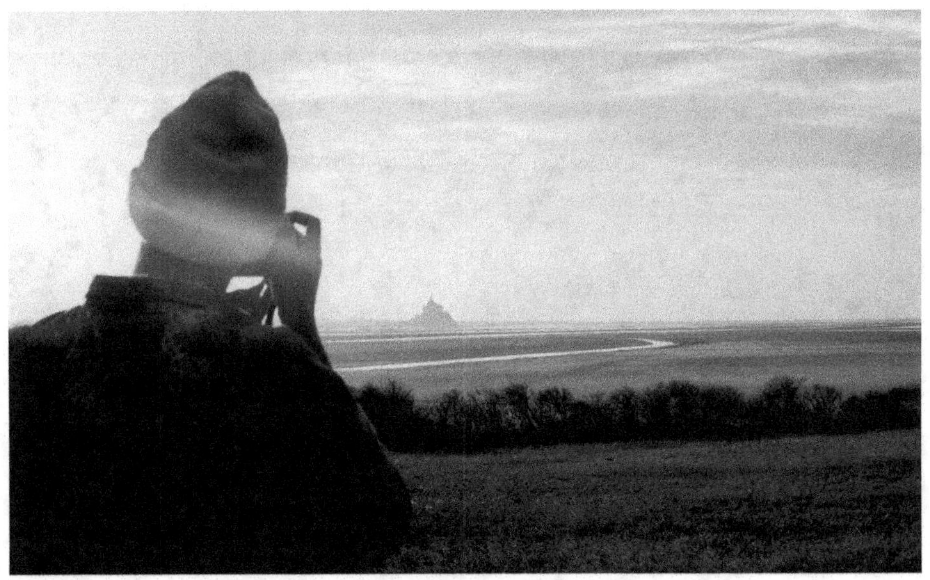

ME: What Do I Have to Do?

- Identify your support system: Who can you rely on for help? Make a list of family members, friends, and community resources.
- Communicate needs clearly: Be open about what you need, whether it's emotional support, practical help, or simply someone to talk to.

MYSELF: Personal Preparation
Caregiving can be emotionally and physically taxing, so it's crucial to prepare yourself for the journey:

Stress Management
Caregiving can be stressful, and managing stress is essential for your well-being. In this eBook, we will cover various stress management techniques, including mindfulness, exercise, and relaxation strategies.

Mental Health
It's important to recognize the impact caregiving can have on your mental health. We'll explore how to maintain emotional balance, seek professional help when needed, and build resilience.

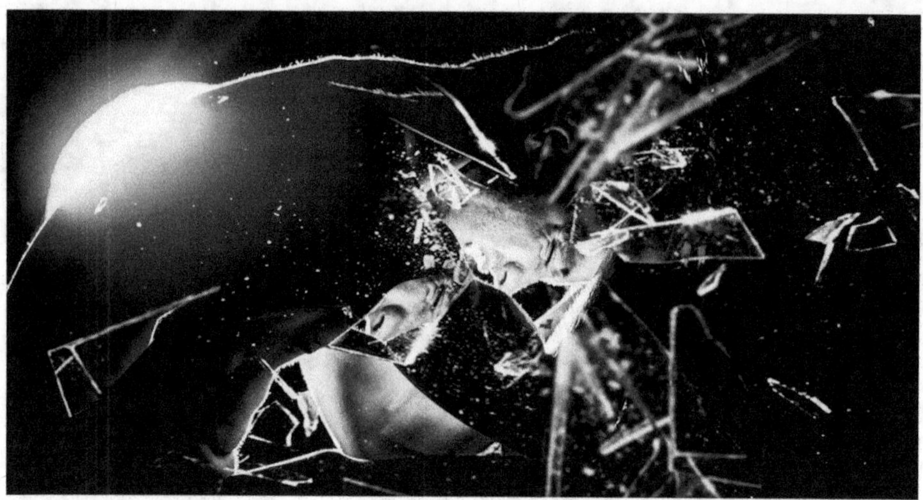

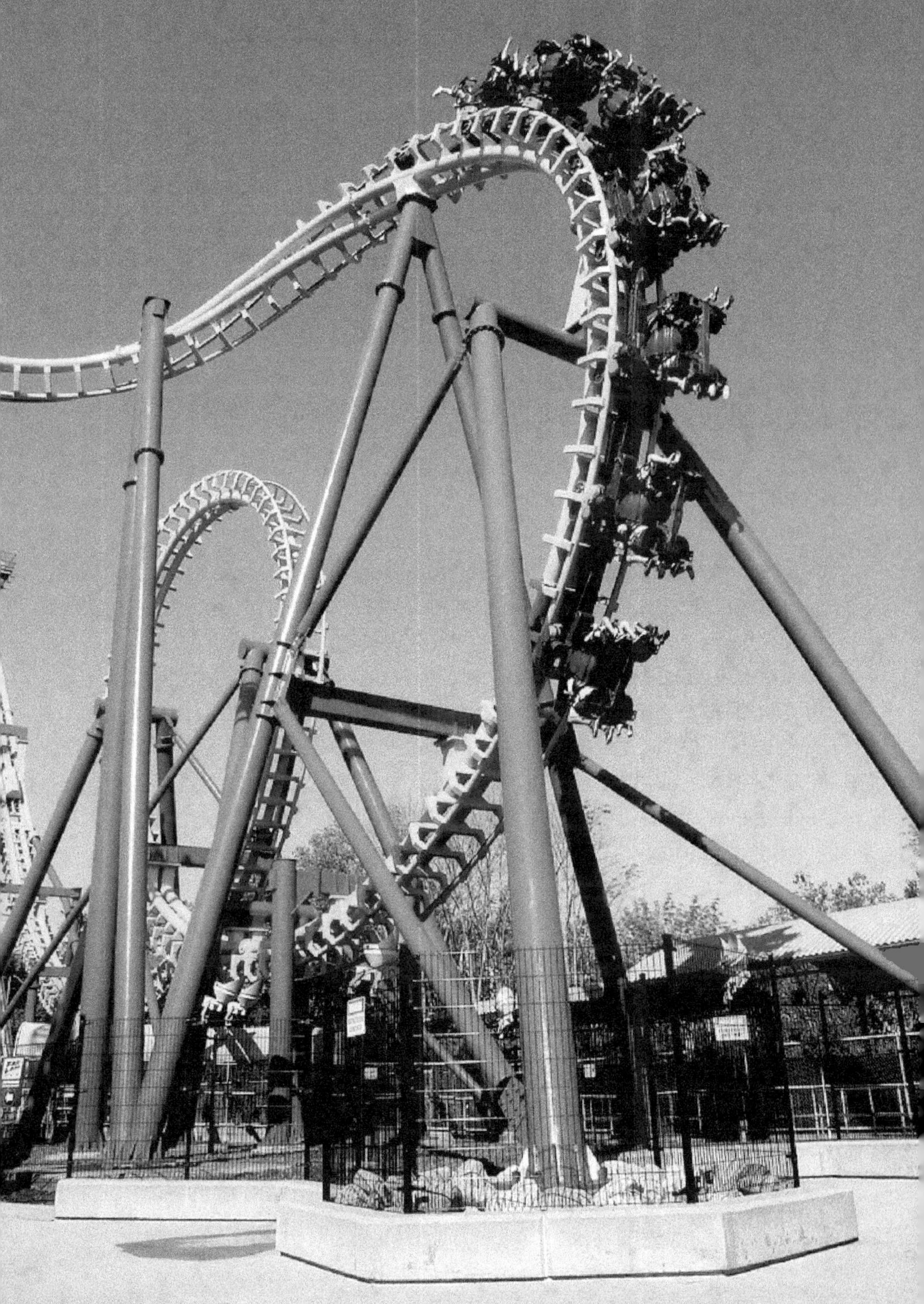

"Life's a rollercoaster"

1.3
Keeping a Sense of Humour

Caregiving is a serious responsibility, filled with challenges and emotional highs and lows. Amidst the seriousness, it's essential to remember the power of humour. Maintaining a sense of humour can be a lifeline, helping to lighten the load and bring moments of joy into your caregiving journey. In this chapter, we'll explore the importance of humour in caregiving and share some practical tips and stories to illustrate how laughter can make a difference.

The Power of Laughter
Laughter is often said to be the best medicine, and there's a lot of truth to that. Here are some of the ways humour and laughter can positively impact both caregivers and care recipients:

- **Reduces Stress:** Laughter triggers the release of endorphins, the body's natural feel-good chemicals. This helps reduce stress and promotes an overall sense of well-being.
- **Strengthens Relationships:** Sharing a laugh can strengthen the bond between caregivers and their loved ones. It can break down barriers and create a sense of camaraderie.
- **Improves Mood:** Humour can lift your spirits and those of your loved one, making the day seem a little brighter and more manageable.
- **Enhances Coping Skills:** Humour provides a different perspective, helping you see challenging situations in a new light and enhancing your ability to cope with them.
- **Physical Benefits:** Laughter releases endorphins, reducing stress and boosting immunity.
- **Enhanced Communication:** Laughter can break down barriers and facilitate communication in caregiving relationships. It creates a relaxed atmosphere where difficult topics can be approached more easily, leading to better understanding and collaboration in providing care.

Finding Humour in Everyday Situations

Finding humour in caregiving might seem difficult, especially during tough times, but it's possible. Here are some ways to incorporate humour into your caregiving routine: Care is sometimes about acting. You have to adapt yourself to the audience and the moment.

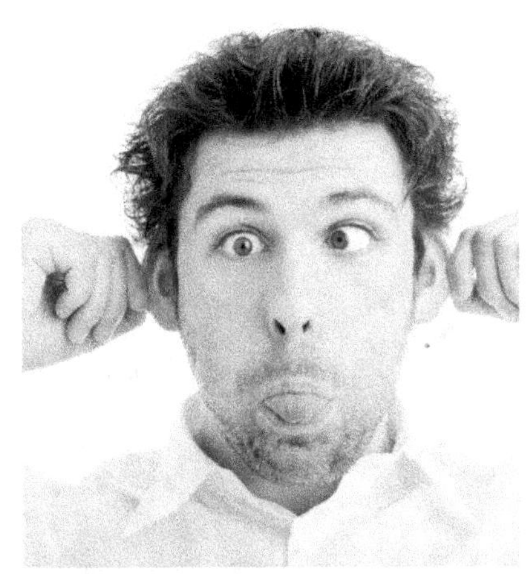

Look for the Light Moments:

Even on the most challenging days, there are often small, funny moments. Keep an eye out for these and allow yourself to laugh at them.

Share Funny Stories:

Swap funny stories with your loved one, other family members, or fellow caregivers. Shared laughter can be a great way to connect and relieve stress.

Watch Comedy Together:

Whether it's a funny movie, TV show, or stand-up comedy special, watching something humorous together can be a delightful break from the routine.

Embrace Silly Moments:

Don't be afraid to be silly. Singing goofy songs, making funny faces, or telling jokes can lighten the mood and make caregiving more enjoyable.

Create A Memory Book

Create a photo album of the good times. I found that this really worked with people and sharing those moments together!

A Personal Story:
The Exploding Catheter Bag

Humour can sometimes find you in the most unexpected and less-than-pleasant situations.

I remember one time when I was caring for a man who had a catheter. While getting him ready, my colleague failed to notice that his leg bag had started to fill up. As we were talking to the man, I suddenly heard a pop. I looked up and saw that the bag had exploded, and my colleague was covered in urine.

Although it wasn't pleasant at the time, we couldn't help but laugh at the absurdity of the situation. That laughter helped us get through the clean-up process with a lighter heart and reminded us that not everything has to be taken so seriously.

Practical Tips for Keeping a Sense of Humour

Here are some practical tips to help you keep a sense of humour in your caregiving journey:

- **Start the Day with a Smile:** Begin your day with something that makes you smile, whether it's a funny video, a comic strip, or a light-hearted conversation.
- **Don't Take Yourself Too Seriously:** Allow yourself to laugh at your own mistakes and imperfections. Caregiving is challenging, and it's okay not to be perfect.
- **Create a Humour Journal:** Keep a journal where you jot down funny moments, quotes, or anecdotes. When you're having a tough day, revisit these entries for a quick pick-me-up.
- **Engage in Playful Activities:** Play games or engage in activities that both you and your loved one enjoy. Board games, card games, or even simple word games can bring laughter and enjoyment.
- **Surround Yourself with Positivity:** Choose to be around people who have a positive outlook and a good sense of humour. Their energy can be contagious and uplifting.

Embracing Humour as a Coping Mechanism

Incorporating humour into your caregiving routine isn't about ignoring the seriousness of the situation or minimizing the challenges. Instead, it's about finding a healthy way to cope with the stress and emotional weight of caregiving. Laughter can be a powerful tool for maintaining your own mental health and creating a more positive environment for your loved one

Conclusion

Keeping a sense of humour in caregiving is not just a nice-to-have; it's a vital coping strategy that can make a significant difference in your daily life. By embracing humour, you can reduce stress, strengthen relationships, and improve your overall well-being. Remember, it's okay to laugh, even when things are tough. Laughter is a reminder that amidst the challenges, there is still joy to be found.

As you continue on your caregiving journey, don't forget to find moments of laughter and lightness. They will help you navigate the ups and downs with a resilient spirit and a smile on your face. Embrace the funny moments, share them with others, and allow humour to be a source of comfort and strength.

Remember to make ME laugh. It will help. Remember to make MYSELF happy as this will help you, and enjoy laughing with THE OTHER ONE. They will feel so much better for it.

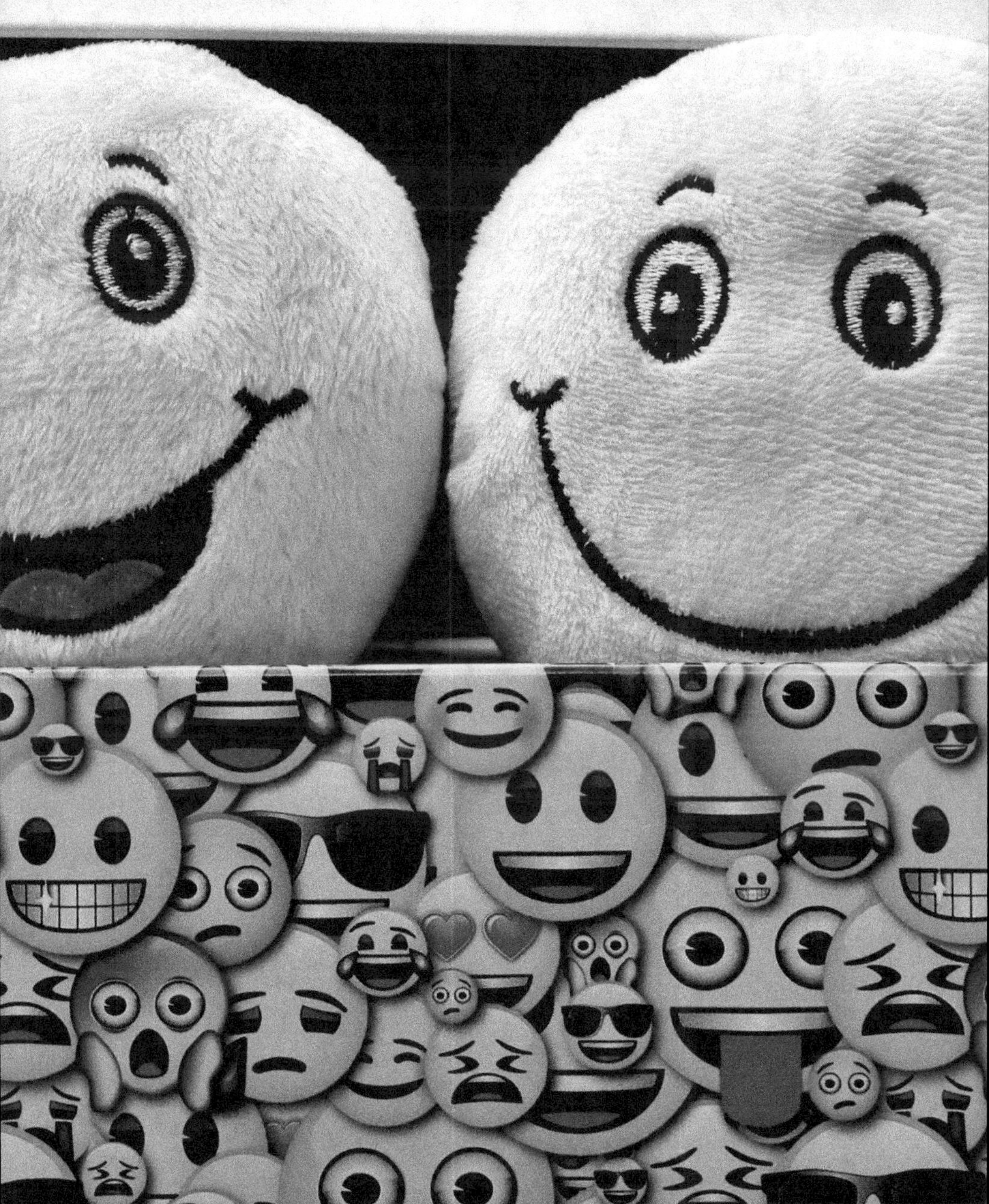
"Finding laughter in life's lows brings light to the darkness."

THE LAUGHING GNOME

In a garden so green, where the flowers do roam, Lived a
small, merry chap called the Laughing Gnome.
With a heart full of cheer and a twinkle in his eye,
He cared for the critters beneath the blue sky.

He'd tend to the birds, the squirrels, and bees,
With a chuckle and grin, putting all at ease.
His laughter was magic, so jolly and bright,
Bringing warmth to the day and joy to the night.

When creatures felt down or were in a fix,
He'd be there to help with his bag full of tricks.
No matter the challenge, no matter the strain,
The Laughing Gnome never would buckle in pain.

With a hop and a skip, he'd come to their aid, Standing
tall with a smile, never afraid.
His spirit unbroken, his heart full of glee,
He'd shout to the shadows, defiant and free:

"Ha Ha Ha, He He He, I'm the Laughing Gnome and you
can't catch me!"

"Inspired By Bowie"

CHAPTER TWO

UNDERSTANDING MENTAL HEALTH IN CARE GIVING

"Even in the midst of challenges, maintaining a positive mindset can light the way to resilience and healing. Embrace the journey, cherish the small victories, and be strong"

2.1
The Emotional Landscape of Caregiving!

This is the heart of caregiving—a journey unlike any other, filled with a spectrum of emotions that can sway from the peaks of joy to the valleys of despair, often all in one day. In this module, I will delve into the diverse emotional experiences that define the caregiving role, acknowledging the highs and lows that shape this profound journey. By the end I hope you will better understand ME, MYSELF and THE OTHER ONE.

The Emotional Spectrum

Imagine Sarah, a devoted daughter caring for her elderly mother with dementia. On good days, Sarah finds laughter and delight in shared moments, like when her mother unexpectedly recalls a cherished family vacation, and they both end up chuckling over a silly incident from the past. Yet, there are also days when Sarah feels the sharp sting of frustration and anger as she repeats instructions for simple tasks, feeling drained by the repetition and the resistance.

Joy and Fulfilment

For many, like Sarah on her good days, caregiving is punctuated with moments of deep fulfilment. These moments can come unexpectedly, like a smile of appreciation or a quiet thank you that reminds caregivers why they've taken on this role. The joy derived from knowing you are providing comfort and support to a loved one is profound and can be deeply affirming.

Frustration and Anger

However, caregiving is not without its trials. The same Sarah who smiles with her mother over fond memories can feel her patience wearing thin as she navigates the complexities of healthcare appointments or manages sudden changes in her mother's behaviour. It's common for caregivers to experience frustration or even anger, emotions that can feel magnified by exhaustion and constant demands.

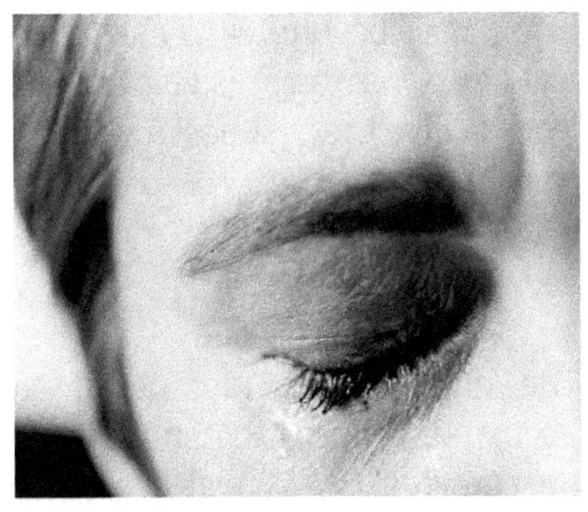

Overwhelm and Being Pulled in All Directions

Feeling overwhelmed is another hallmark of the caregiving experience. Caregivers often report feeling as if they are being pulled in multiple directions, struggling to balance the needs of their loved one with personal and professional responsibilities. This can lead to a sense of being lost in a sea of tasks, where the shore seems just out of reach.

Grief and Loss

Amid these challenges, there is also space for grief. Caregivers like Sarah must often mourn the loss of the person they once knew even while they care for them. This grief can be confusing and isolating, a continual goodbye to pieces of a beloved's personality and independence.

Laughter and Lightness Yet, it's important to remember that caregiving also offers unique opportunities for laughter and lightness. These moments, though sometimes fleeting, are vital. They serve as a reminder that even in the midst of caregiving, there can be instances of joy and levity that buoy both the caregiver and the recipient.

When You May Have to Let Go

Perhaps one of the most heart-wrenching aspects of caregiving is recognizing when home care is no longer the best option. Making the decision to move a loved one into a care facility can evoke a complex mix of relief, guilt, sorrow, and acceptance. It is a profound emotional shift, acknowledging that your loved one needs a level of professional care that is beyond what can be provided at home. This transition can feel like a loss, yet it is also an act of love and responsibility, ensuring they receive the best possible care.

Conclusion

The emotional landscape of caregiving is complex and varied. Recognizing and understanding these emotions is crucial, not only for the caregivers' own health but also for the quality of care they provide. If you let it take over in a negative way , it will infect MYSELF and THE OTHER ONE. In the coming chapters, we will explore strategies for navigating these emotional terrains. By preparing to manage these feelings effectively, caregivers can ensure that they are supporting their loved ones while also taking care of themselves. Remember, acknowledging these emotions as part of your caregiving journey is the first step towards a healthier, more balanced caregiving experience.

2.2
Common Mental Health Challenges for Caregivers!

Introduction

Caring for a loved one is not just physically demanding; it's also a mental marathon. In this module, we delve into the common mental health challenges that caregivers face. While caregiving can be incredibly rewarding, the emotional toll it takes is real and significant. Understanding these challenges is the first step toward managing them effectively and maintaining your well-being.

Stress and Anxiety

Stress is perhaps the most universal experience among caregivers. The constant pressure of caregiving responsibilities, coupled with concerns for the future, can lead to chronic stress and anxiety. Symptoms might include restlessness, irritability, muscle tension, and difficulty concentrating. Chronic stress can not only wear you down mentally but can also lead to serious physical health issues, such as heart disease and a weakened immune system.

Depression

Many caregivers experience periods of sadness, but when feelings of despair and hopelessness persist, it may indicate depression. This mental health condition is characterized by significant changes in mood, behaviour, and physical functions—such as sleep, appetite, and energy levels. Depression in caregivers can often go unrecognized and untreated because they may attribute these feelings to the normal stress of caregiving and not recognize the severity of their condition.

Burnout.
Burnout is a state of emotional, physical, and mental exhaustion caused by excessive and prolonged stress. It occurs when you feel overwhelmed, emotionally drained, and unable to meet constant demands. As the stress continues, you begin to lose the interest and motivation that led you to take on a caregiving role in the first place. Burnout reduces productivity and saps your energy, leaving you feeling increasingly helpless, hopeless, cynical, and resentful.

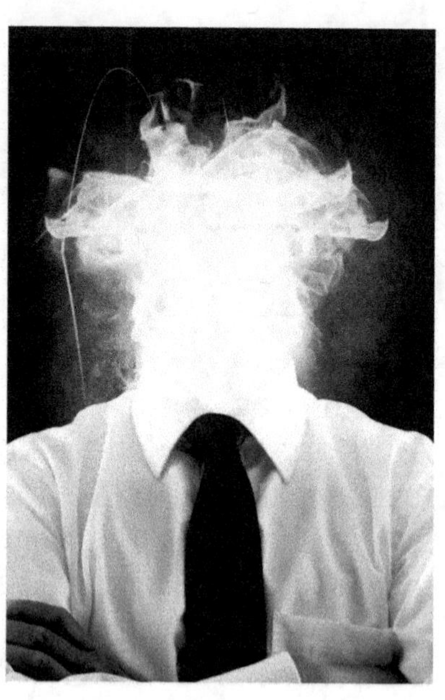

Isolation and Loneliness

Caregivers often find themselves feeling isolated or cut off from others. This isolation can stem from the relentless demands of caregiving, which can make it difficult to maintain friendships or participate in social activities. Over time, isolation can lead to loneliness, which is associated with increased risks of mental health issues like depression and anxiety. It's important for caregivers to seek support from community groups or online forums to mitigate these feelings.

Guilt

 Guilt is a frequent companion to caregiving. Caregivers may feel guilty for not doing enough, not providing care perfectly, or for feeling resentful towards their caregiving responsibilities. This guilt can be compounded by external pressures and societal expectations about what caregiving should look like. Recognizing that no one is a perfect caregiver is vital. Accepting that you are doing the best you can in a challenging situation is crucial to overcoming guilt.

Conclusion

Addressing these common mental health challenges is essential not only for your health but also for the quality of care you provide. The subsequent modules will offer strategies for managing these challenges, emphasizing the importance of self-care and seeking support when needed. By acknowledging and addressing these mental health challenges, caregivers can find more strength and resilience in their caregiving journey, ultimately leading to better outcomes for both them and those they care for.

A famous line I always turn when I need cheering is from a famous Monty Python's song:

"ALWAYS LOOK ON THE BRIGHT SIDE OF LIFE!"

This line is part of the song's chorus and is featured in the movie Monty Python's Life of Brian. The song, written by Eric Idle, is known for its upbeat melody and ironic lyrics that encourage a positive outlook even in dire circumstances.

This is the song I want played at my funeral!

2.3
Recognising Mental Health in THE OTHER ONE!

Introduction

Caring for someone with mental health issues presents unique challenges for caregivers. Unlike physical ailments, mental health conditions can be less visible and harder to detect, making it crucial for caregivers to be vigilant and observant. In this module, we'll explore common mental health issues in care recipients, how they can manifest behaviourally, and the importance of recognizing and addressing them promptly.

The Complexity of Mental Health Conditions

Navigating the landscape of mental health conditions presents a multifaceted challenge for caregivers. These conditions encompass a diverse array of disorders, ranging from anxiety and depression to more complex neurological conditions like dementia, autism, acquired brain injury, and various learning difficulties. Each condition manifests uniquely, with its own set of symptoms and behavioural patterns. Imagine the labyrinth of challenges faced by caregivers when dealing with conditions where the very essence of cognition is altered. Conditions like dementia can unravel memories and disorient perceptions, while autism can distort social interactions and communication. Acquired brain injuries can disrupt cognitive function, leading to a profound shift in personality and behaviour. In the midst of this complexity, caregivers must navigate the nuances of each condition, adapting their caregiving approach to meet the specific needs of their loved ones. Locked away within the labyrinth of their condition, individuals may find themselves adrift in a sea of confusion and uncertainty, their minds tethered to a reality that eludes comprehension. For caregivers, unravelling this complexity requires patience, empathy, and a deep understanding of the intricacies of mental health conditions.

Behavioural Manifestations

One of the primary challenges caregivers face is recognizing mental health issues through their loved one's behaviours. Mental health conditions can manifest in various ways, including changes in mood, cognition, and behaviour. For example, a person with depression may exhibit symptoms such as persistent sadness, loss of interest in previously enjoyed activities, changes in appetite or sleep patterns, and feelings of worthlessness or guilt.

Impact on Behaviours

The nature of mental health conditions can significantly impact a care recipient's behaviours, making caregiving more challenging. For instance, someone with dementia may experience confusion, agitation, aggression, or wandering, while those with schizophrenia may have hallucinations or delusions. These behaviours can be distressing for both the care recipient and the caregiver, requiring patience, understanding, and specialized strategies to manage effectively.

Recognizing Signs and Symptoms

Recognizing signs and symptoms of mental health issues requires careful observation and communication. Pay attention to changes in behaviour, mood, and daily functioning, and don't hesitate to seek professional guidance if you notice anything concerning. Keep in mind that some behaviours may be subtle or easily dismissed, so trust your instincts and advocate for your loved one's well-being.

Seeking Professional Help

When it comes to mental health issues, early intervention is key. If you suspect that your loved one is experiencing mental health challenges, don't hesitate to seek professional help. Consult with their healthcare provider or a mental health specialist who can conduct a thorough assessment and recommend appropriate treatment options. Remember that you don't have to navigate this journey alone—there are resources and support available to help you and your loved one through this challenging time.

Example: Recognizing Depression in a Care Recipient

Let's consider the case of Jack, who has been caring for his elderly father, George, who recently lost his spouse. Over the past few weeks, Jack has noticed changes in George's behaviour.

He seems withdrawn, lacks interest in his favourite activities, and struggles to sleep at night. George's appetite has also decreased, and he frequently expresses feelings of sadness and hopelessness. Recognizing these signs, Jack reaches out to George's doctor, who confirms that George is experiencing depression and recommends counselling and medication.

Conclusion

Recognizing mental health issues in care recipients demands unwavering vigilance, deep empathy, and clear communication. It's crucial to understand that the individual's condition, whether it be autism, dementia, learning difficulties, or something like MS, may exacerbate their confusion, feelings of helplessness, or inability to comprehend their situation. Caregivers must not only identify these challenges but also actively collaborate with the individual, if possible, to alleviate their distress.

This collaborative approach involves engaging in open dialogue, validating their emotions, and working together to find coping mechanisms that suit their unique needs. It's about creating a safe space where the care recipient feels heard, understood, and empowered to participate in their own care journey. By fostering a sense of agency and autonomy, caregivers can help alleviate feelings of anxiety and uncertainty, promoting a more positive and empowering caregiving experience for both parties.

Furthermore, caregivers should actively seek out resources and support networks tailored to the specific mental health challenges their loved one is facing. This may involve connecting with mental health professionals, attending support groups, or accessing community services that offer specialized care and assistance.

In the upcoming modules, we will delve into effective strategies for supporting care recipients with diverse mental health challenges. From implementing personalized care plans to integrating therapeutic activities into daily routines, we will explore a range of approaches aimed at fostering a nurturing and supportive caregiving environment that prioritizes holistic well-being.

This journey is akin to almost relearning about THE OTHER ONE, understanding their unique needs and challenges anew, and embarking on a collaborative path towards improved mental health and overall well-being.

WHEN LOIS LANE BECAME SUPERGIRL

In Metropolis, Superman was brave and grand,
Known for his strength and a steady hand.
But time moved on, even for the Man of Steel,
He forgot things, his memory started to reel.

Lois Lane, his love, now had a new task,
Caring for Clark, behind the hero's mask.
One morning, he tried to put on his tights,
But over his head, giving Lois delights.

"Clark, my dear, tights are for your legs," she said,
Laughing as she helped him, shaking her head.
He smiled, confused but bright in his gaze,
"Are you sure? They make quite a hat these days!"

Despite all the challenges, Lois would stay,
Even when his powers caused disarray.
He toasted bread with his heat vision beam,
"Clark, lightly toasted, not a smoky dream!"

And when he forgot his strength in a flash,
Groceries launched with a powerful smash.
"Oh well," she sighed, with a loving grin,
"We'll have our salad another day, my kin."

Clark's grand gestures, so sweet and divine,
He'd fly for croissants but bring back a sign.
"Bagels from Brooklyn?" Lois would jest,
"It's the thought that counts, you always do your best."

One day, he flew off to save a small cat,
But instead of a feline, returned with a hat.
He aimed to face Lex, the bald villain's dread,
Yet somehow ended up smashing an egg instead.

Through all the confusion, with laughter and love,
Clark would look at her, like a gift from above.
"Lois, you are my hero," he'd say with delight,
In those precious moments, everything felt right.

For it didn't matter if he forgot his name,
Lois remembered, and loved him just the same.
With or without tights, in each other's embrace,
Their love soared high, in every tender trace.

So Lois the Carer became the true hero,
Looking after Superman, her heart a warm glow.
In the end, it was love that truly defined,
Their legendary bond, forever intertwined.

CHAPTER 3

DO I REALLY HAVE TO DO THAT!

"I didn't realize I had to do that! But hey, who knew I'd become a jack-of-all-trades, from fashion designer to diplomat, all before my morning coffee!"

3.1 Counsellor, Diplomat, Entertainer, Cleaner, and the Doer of Everything

Introduction

Entering the world of caregiving often means wearing many hats. From providing emotional support to performing daily household tasks, caregivers take on a multitude of roles that can sometimes feel overwhelming. In this module, we will explore the various roles you may find yourself in and offer strategies to manage these responsibilities effectively.

The Many Hats of a Caregiver

Counsellor

As a caregiver, you often become the primary source of emotional support for your loved one. This role requires patience, empathy, and excellent listening skills. Your loved one might need someone to talk to about their fears, frustrations, and experiences. Here are some tips for being an effective counsellor:

- **Listen Actively**: Give your full attention, acknowledge their feelings, and avoid interrupting.

- **Paraphrase Back**: Repeat the key points back to the person you are spreaking to. This reassures them that you are listening.

- **Offer Reassurance:** Provide comfort and encouragement, letting them know they are not alone. Never judge them.

- **Seek Professional Help:** Recognize when professional counselling might be needed and help facilitate access to these services.

Entertainer

Keeping your loved one engaged and entertained is crucial for their mental and emotional well-being. This role can involve finding activities that they enjoy, organizing social interactions, and keeping their mind active. Here are some ideas:

- **Create a Schedule:** Plan daily activities such as puzzles, games, reading, or watching favourite movies.

- **Encourage Hobbies:** Support their interests and hobbies, whether it's gardening, knitting, or painting.

- **Social Interaction:** Arrange visits with friends and family or join community groups that offer activities for individuals with similar conditions.

Cleaner

Maintaining a clean and safe environment is essential for the health and comfort of your loved one. This role includes regular cleaning, laundry, and ensuring that the living space is free of hazards. Here are some strategies to manage cleaning tasks:

- **Set a Routine:** Establish a cleaning schedule to keep the home tidy and organized.

- **Prioritize Tasks:** Focus on areas that need the most attention, such as the kitchen, bathroom, and living areas.

- **Seek Help:** Don't hesitate to ask for help from family members or consider hiring a cleaning service if needed.

Gardener

Maintaining a pleasant and therapeutic environment can involve gardening. This role includes taking care of outdoor spaces and possibly involving your loved one in light gardening activities.

There is something therapeutic about gardening that people enjoy. Either the labour of digging or weeding, or the growing of flowers and seeing the pleasure of wildlife going about there business. It could be the productive part of producing vegetable and enjoying the bounties of your labour on your plate.

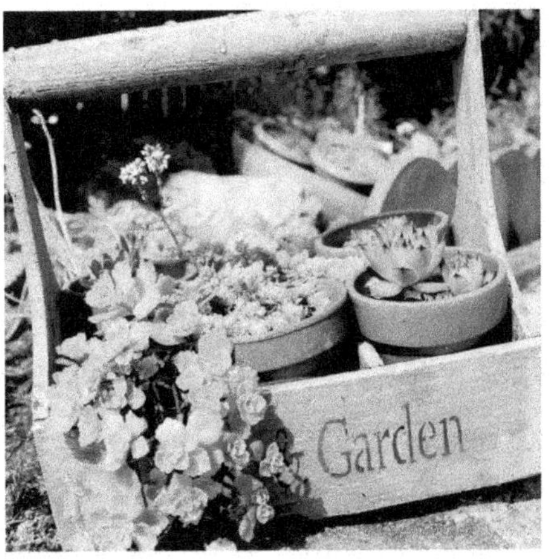

This is an activity you can do with THE OTHER ONE. Here's how to manage this:

- **Create a Safe Space:** Ensure the garden is accessible and free of hazards.

- **Involve Your Loved One:** Gardening can be a fun activity that your loved one might enjoy.

- **Simplicity is Key:** Choose low-maintenance plants and gardening techniques to keep it manageable.

Financial Expert

Managing finances is a critical aspect of caregiving. This role involves budgeting, paying bills, managing insurance claims, and possibly handling your loved one's financial affairs. Here are some tips:

- **Create a Budget:** Track all income and expenses to ensure you stay within budget.

- **Monitor Accounts:** Regularly review bank statements and financial records to catch any discrepancies.

- **Seek Professional Advice:** Consider consulting a financial advisor to help manage complex financial matters.

Fashion Designer

Ensuring that your loved one is comfortably and appropriately dressed can boost their morale and dignity. This role involves selecting suitable clothing, helping with dressing, and sometimes making or altering clothes. Here's how to approach it:

- **Comfort First:** Choose clothing that is easy to put on and take off, and comfortable to wear.

- **Adapt to Needs**: Modify clothing to accommodate medical devices or physical limitations.

- **Boost Confidence:** Pick outfits that your loved one likes and that make them feel good about themselves.

Diplomat

As a caregiver, you often find yourself in the role of a diplomat, navigating complex relationships and acting as a mediator between your loved one, family members, and healthcare professionals. This role can be a source of many arguments, feelings of frustration, and even grief. It requires excellent communication and negotiation skills to keep the peace and ensure everyone is on the same page.. Here are some strategies:

- **Establish Open Lines of Communication:** Make sure that everyone involved in your loved one's care understands the care plan and their specific roles. Regular family meetings or group calls can help keep everyone informed and aligned.

- **Manage Conflicts:** Address disagreements calmly and seek solutions that consider everyone's needs.

- **Advocate:** Speak up for your loved one's needs and preferences in medical settings.

- **Be Transparent:** Share updates honestly and openly. Keeping everyone in the loop prevents misunderstandings and fosters trust.

Nurse

Providing medical care is a significant part of caregiving. This includes managing medications, giving medication at the correct times, attending medical appointments, and handling medical equipment. Here's how to approach this role:

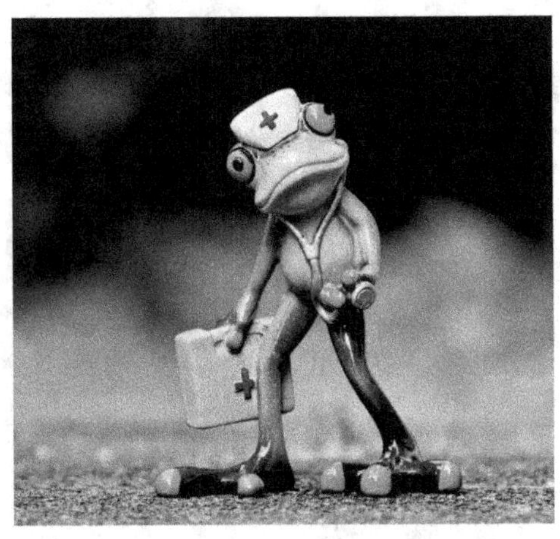

In care we have something called the 7 R's. (Can also be 6 or 8 but these are the important ones.): Carers follow this when managing and giving medication.

Right Person: Make sure it is their medication you are giving, not someone elses or yours!
Right Time: Make sure it's being given at the right time of day.
Right Dose: Don't get your litres confused with your millilitres.
Right Route: You don't chew a suppository do you?
Right Medication: Make sure it's the right medication. Medication names can be similar, often from latin and are difficult to pronounce.
The Right to Refuse: People have human rights.
Right Documentation: Don't forget to write it down they have taken it. It's easy to forget and give again!

Other approaches are:

- **Stay Informed:** Learn about your loved one's medical conditions and treatment plans.

- **Medication Management:** Keep an organized schedule of medications and dosages.

- **Emergency Preparedness:** Know how to handle medical emergencies and keep contact information for healthcare providers readily available.

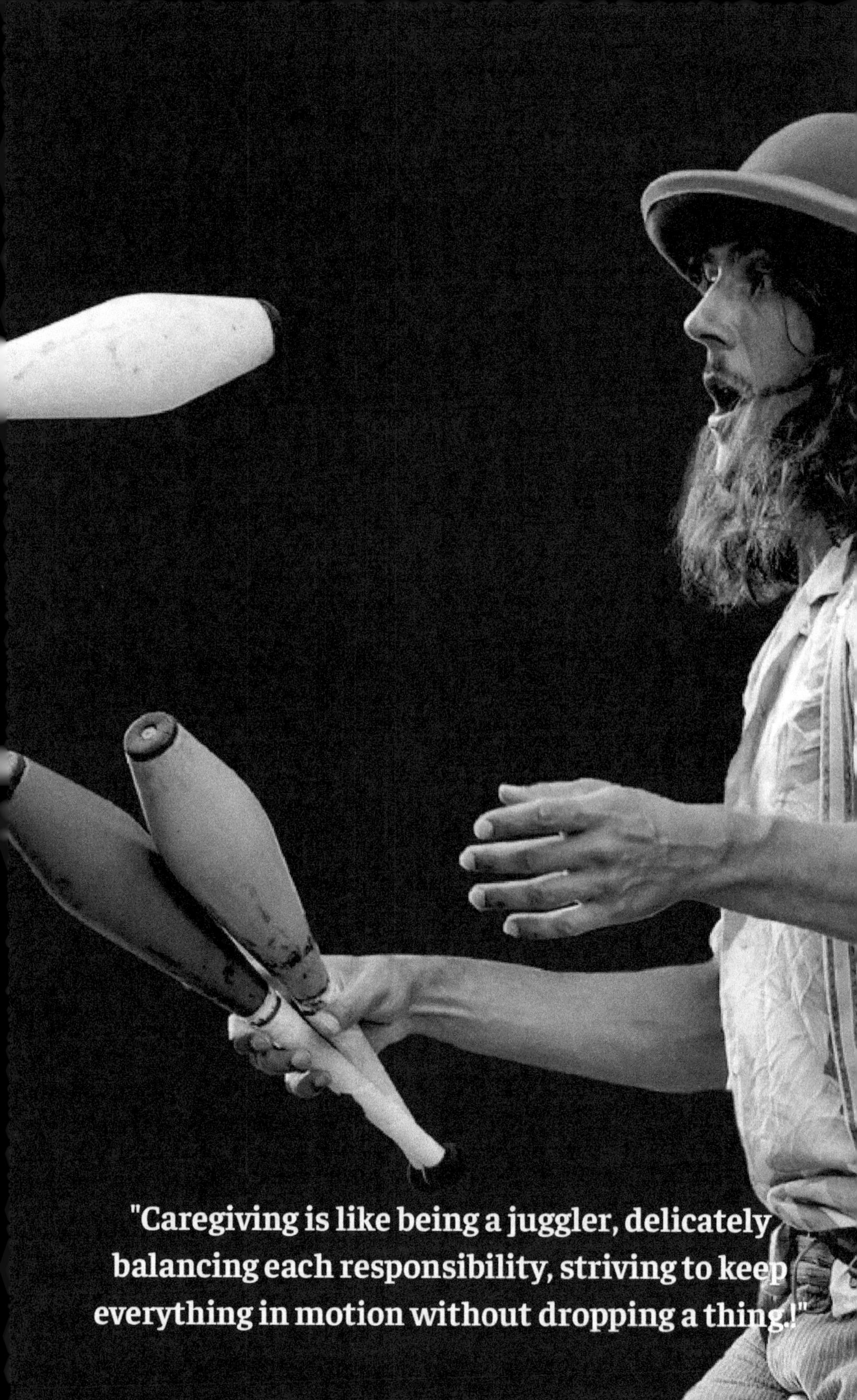
"Caregiving is like being a juggler, delicately balancing each responsibility, striving to keep everything in motion without dropping a thing!"

Do-er of Everything!

As a caregiver, you often become the "do-er of everything," managing various tasks that ensure the smooth functioning of daily life. This can include grocery shopping, cooking, managing medications, and more. Here are some ways to handle this role:

- **Stay Organized:** Use planners, calendars, and to-do lists to keep track of tasks and appointments.

- **Delegate Responsibilities:** Involve other family members or friends in caregiving tasks to share the load.

- **Simplify Tasks:** Look for ways to simplify or streamline tasks, such as meal prepping or using delivery services for groceries and medications.

- **Keep a Journal:** Write Everything down. It is proof of what an amazing job you have been doing. It can help when you may need extra funding.

Conclusion

Wearing many hats as a caregiver is a challenging yet rewarding experience. By understanding the various roles you play and implementing strategies to manage these responsibilities, you can provide the best possible care for your loved one while maintaining your own health and well-being. Remember, it's important to seek support and take care of yourself as you navigate this journey. It is also important that you do this with the person. In care you hear about person centred care. This means the person is at the heart of everything that is done. With preparation, organization, and a positive attitude, you can embrace the multifaceted role of a caregiver and make a meaningful difference in your loved one's life.

Now read onto the next section as there is an important part of care giving that we need to mention, and YES, ME may have to do this with THE OTHER ONE.

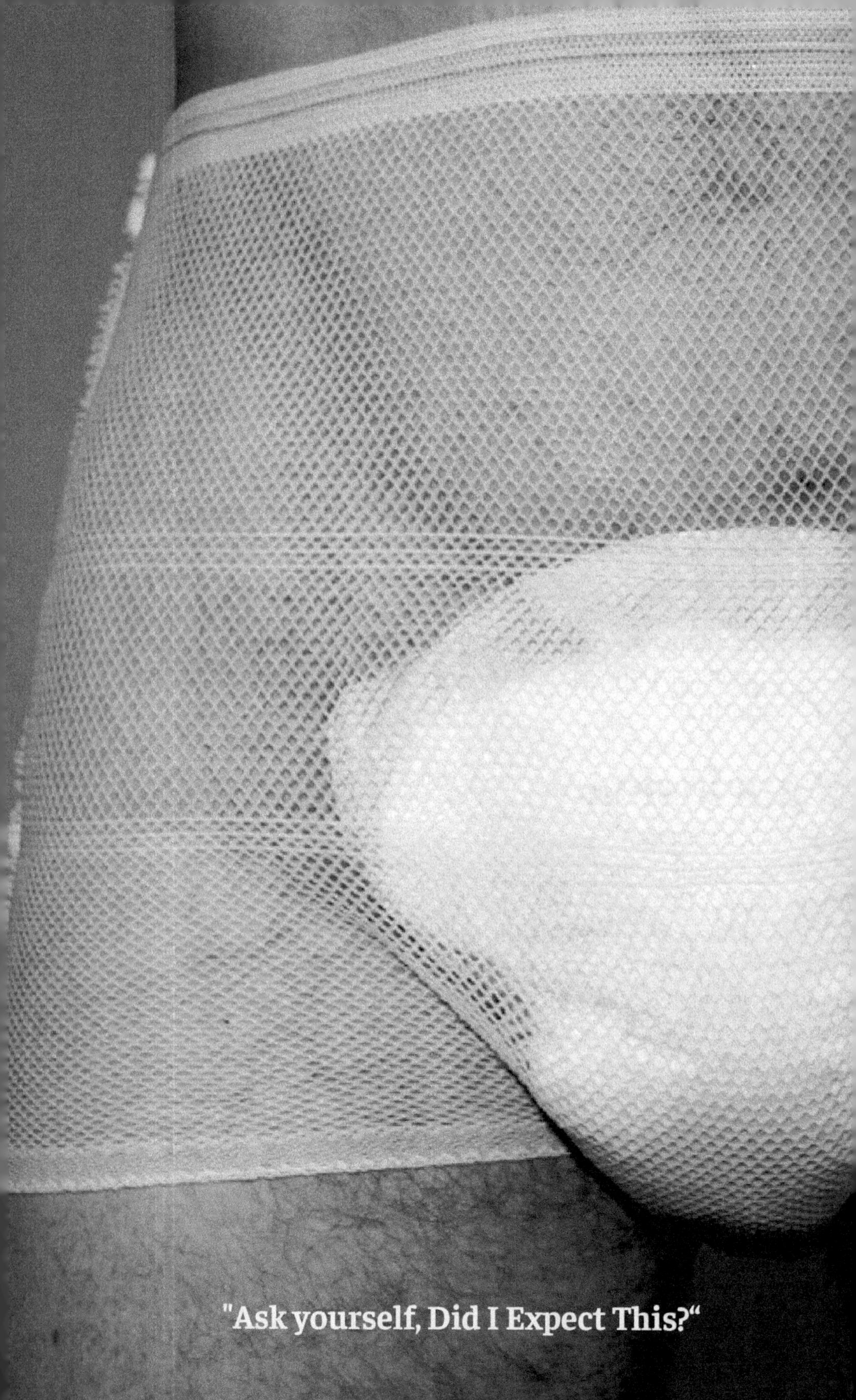

"Ask yourself, Did I Expect This?"

3.2
Poo, All- Personal Care and Dignity.

Introduction

I don't wish to sugar coat things, so this section is about the harsh realities of personal care. It is important that you know what to expect. Caring for a loved one often involves tasks that are deeply personal and intimate. Providing personal care can be challenging, particularly when it involves cleaning and handling bodily fluids. However, it is essential to approach these tasks with dignity and respect, using the right terminology and maintaining a compassionate attitude.

Understanding Personal Care

Personal care encompasses a wide range of activities, including:

- **Cleaning Bottoms**: Whether due to incontinence or illness, you may need to clean your loved one after they use the toilet.

- **Handling Genitals:** This can include cleaning penises and vaginas, which requires sensitivity and respect.

- **Managing Incontinence:** This often involves changing adult pads, which in the UK are referred to as pads rather than nappies or diapers.

- **Dealing with Vomit:** Cleaning up vomit can be particularly unpleasant but is sometimes necessary.

- **Handling Urine:** Managing urinary incontinence includes cleaning up spills and changing wet clothes or bed linens.

Types of Other Personal Care:
Personal care tasks can include:

Bathing or Showering
Bathing or showering involves assisting your loved one in maintaining personal hygiene by cleansing their body. This task may include:

- **Assisting with Undressing:** Helping your loved one remove their clothing before entering the bath or shower.

- **Assisting with Washing:** Helping your loved one wash their body using soap and water, ensuring thorough cleansing.

- **Assisting with Drying:** Helping your loved one dry off after bathing or showering to prevent skin irritation or discomfort.

- **Assisting with Dressing:** Helping your loved one get dressed in clean clothes after bathing or showering.

Dressing and Grooming:
Dressing and grooming involve helping your loved one select appropriate clothing and maintain their personal appearance. This task may include:

- **Assisting with Clothing Selection:** Helping your loved one choose clothing that is suitable for the weather and occasion.

- **Assisting with Dressing:** Helping your loved one put on and fasten clothing, including buttons, zippers, and shoelaces.

- **Assisting with Hair Care:** Helping your loved one brush or style their hair, or assisting with shaving or trimming facial hair if needed.

- **Assisting with Personal Care Products:** Helping your loved one apply personal care products such as lotion, deodorant, or perfume.

Types of Other Personal Care:

Oral Hygiene

Oral hygiene involves helping your loved one maintain a healthy mouth and teeth. This task may include:

- **Assisting with Brushing Teeth:** Helping your loved one brush their teeth using a toothbrush and toothpaste, ensuring thorough cleaning.

- **Assisting with Denture Care:** Helping your loved one remove, clean, and replace dentures if applicable.

- **Assisting with Mouth Care:** Helping your loved one rinse their mouth with mouthwash or water, or assisting with flossing if needed.

According to NICE, more than half of older adults who live in care homes have tooth decay, compared to 40% of over 75s who do not live in care homes.

Toileting

Toileting involves assisting your loved one with using the toilet and maintaining continence. This task may include:

- **Assisting with Transferring:** Helping your loved one transfer to and from the toilet safely if mobility is a concern.

- **Assisting with Personal Hygiene:** Helping your loved one wipe themselves after using the toilet if needed, ensuring cleanliness.

- **Assisting with Incontinence Products:** Helping your loved one use and change incontinence products such as pads or briefs if necessary.

Incontinence Care

Incontinence care involves managing urinary or fecal incontinence to maintain cleanliness and prevent skin irritation. This task may include:

- **Assisting with Cleaning:** Helping your loved one clean themselves after an episode of incontinence, ensuring thorough cleansing.

- **Assisting with Incontinence Products:** Helping your loved one use and change incontinence products such as pads, briefs, or bed pads as needed.

- **Assisting with Skin Protection:** Applying barrier creams or ointments to protect the skin from moisture and irritation.

Skin Care

Skin care involves maintaining the health and integrity of your loved one's skin. This task may include:

- **Assisting with Bathing:** Ensuring thorough cleansing during bathing to remove sweat, dirt, and bacteria from the skin.

- **Assisting with Moisturizing:** Applying moisturizing lotion or cream to keep the skin hydrated and prevent dryness or itching.

- **Assisting with Skin Inspection:** Checking the skin regularly for signs of redness, irritation, or pressure sores, and taking appropriate action if needed.

Nail Care

Nail care involves keeping your loved one's nails clean and trimmed to prevent infection and discomfort. This task may include:

- **Assisting with Nail Trimming: Trimming** your loved one's fingernails and toenails carefully using nail clippers or scissors, taking care to avoid cutting the skin.

- **Assisting with Nail Cleaning:** Cleaning underneath the nails to remove dirt and debris, ensuring good hygiene.

Terminology Matters

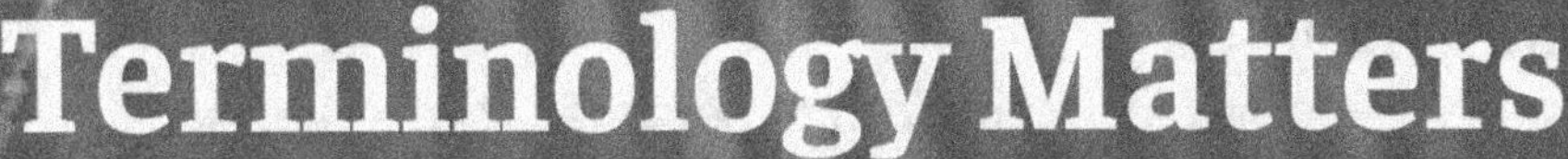

Using appropriate terminology is crucial to maintain dignity and respect:

- **Adult Pads**, Not Nappies/Diapers: In the UK, we use the term "adult pads" instead of "nappies" or "diapers." This distinction helps preserve the dignity of the person receiving care.
- **Leg Bags:** Don't call them Urine bags, Wee bags or Pissy Bags. This is not dignified language to use.
- **Respectful Language**: Use respectful language when referring to body parts and bodily functions. This can make a significant difference in how your loved one feels about the care they receive.

Getting Hands-On

When it comes to providing personal care, I have always recommended it's best to dive in and get hands-on experience as quickly as possible.

Here's why:

- **Overcoming Hesitation:** The thought of cleaning up bodily fluids can be daunting, especially for first-time carers. However, facing these tasks head-on helps build confidence and competence.

- **Dealing with Smells:** Smells can be a significant barrier. Wearing gloves and using scented sprays or masks can help. Over time, you will become more accustomed to the odours.

- **Comparing to Childcare:** Many people assume that because they have changed a baby's nappy, they can handle adult personal care. The reality is different. Adult bodies are larger, often wrinkled, hairier, and come in all shapes and sizes. Understanding this difference can help set realistic expectations.

Empowering Independence

Empowering your loved one to do as much for themselves as possible is crucial for maintaining their dignity and independence. Encourage them to:

- **Participate in Personal Care:** Involve your loved one in their personal care routine as much as possible. This can include tasks like brushing their teeth, combing their hair, or washing their face.

- **Use Adaptive Equipment:** Explore the use of adaptive equipment such as grab bars, shower chairs, or long-handled sponges to make personal care tasks easier and safer for your loved one.

- **Practice Self-Care:** Encourage your loved one to practice self-care activities that promote independence and well-being, such as dressing themselves or using the toilet independently.

The Emotional Aspect
Providing personal care can be emotionally challenging. It is important to:

- **Acknowledge Your Feelings:** It is normal to feel discomfort or unease initially. Acknowledge these feelings and give yourself grace.

- **Seek Support:** Talk to other caregivers or join a support group. Sharing experiences can provide reassurance and practical tips.

- **Stay Positive:** Focus on the positive impact you are having on your loved one's quality of life.

- **It can Feel Strange:** This is natural. You may find that you are caring for a mother. She was the one who brought you into this world. She cared for you as a child and young adult. Now it's your turn to care for her.

Ask Yourself Again!
Can you handle Poo even when sometimes it can go everywhere?

Conclusion

By embracing the reality of personal care tasks and approaching them with respect and professionalism, you can provide the best possible care for your loved one. Remember, every act of care you provide, no matter how small, contributes to their dignity and well-being.

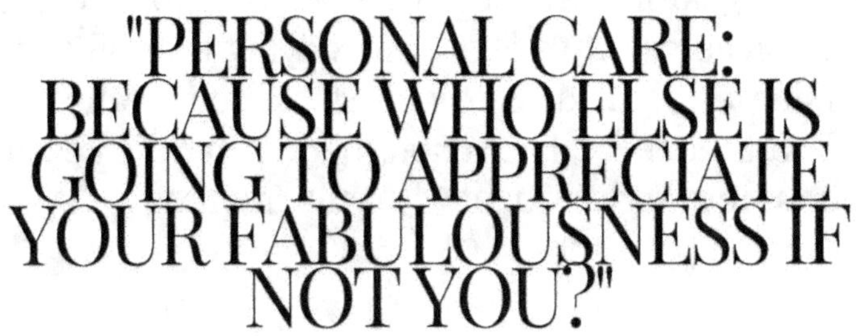

3.3
Guardian Angels.

In the realm of caregiving, every individual is bestowed with a sacred duty: safeguarding. It's not merely a bureaucratic checkbox; it's a lifeline for the vulnerable. Allow me, your guardian angel, to illuminate the significance of this role.

Safeguarding

Safeguarding stands as the fortress against horrors like exploitation, abuse, and neglect. Consider the chilling saga of Winterbourne View, a care home where vulnerable residents were subjected to unspeakable abuse. Shocking reports revealed residents being hit, verbally abused, and even pinned under chairs by those entrusted with their care. This tragic tale serves as a stark reminder that safeguarding breaches can occur anywhere, even within the supposed sanctity of a care setting. But let's not forget, such atrocities could transpire within the walls of a home too.

You Have A Duty Of Care

Every individual, whether a caregiver, family member, or concerned citizen, bears the weighty responsibility of detecting signs of distress, intervening decisively, and championing the rights of those under our watch. Our vigilance serves as the frontline defense against calamity and affords sanctuary to the defenseless.

Remember, safeguarding isn't just a chore; it's a moral obligation that transcends bureaucracy. It's about embodying the spirit of care and ensuring that every individual, regardless of circumstance, is shielded from harm. So, heed this call to action, for every act of safeguarding is a beacon of hope in a world fraught with vulnerability.

Reporting

Reporting suspected abuse is paramount in ensuring the safety and well-being of vulnerable individuals. If you witness or are informed of any form of abuse, it is crucial to document the facts accurately and promptly report them to the appropriate authorities. In the UK, concerns can be reported to local authorities, social services, or safeguarding teams.

In the USA, individuals can contact Adult Protective Services (APS) or Child Protective Services (CPS) depending on the age of the victim. In Canada, concerns can be reported to local child welfare agencies or adult protective services. In Australia, individuals can contact the relevant state or territory department responsible for child protection or adult safeguarding.

Regardless of location, reporting abuse ensures that necessary interventions are made to protect the vulnerable and hold perpetrators accountable, thereby upholding the principles of justice and safeguarding for all.

Remember Simon from Earlier?

Remember Simon from earlier? After needing full-time care, he moved to a supported living service. Unfortunately, he experienced a distressing incident where a carer stole money from him. Encountering any form of abuse, whether it's financial, emotional, or physical, can evoke feelings of anger, sadness, and shock.

It's crucial to remain calm and composed in such situations, as reacting impulsively can escalate the issue further. Instead, take a deep breath, gather your thoughts, and address the situation calmly and assertively. Documenting any incidents and reporting them to the appropriate authorities is essential to ensure the safety and well-being of your loved one and prevent further harm.

Be a Guardian Angel and Show You Care

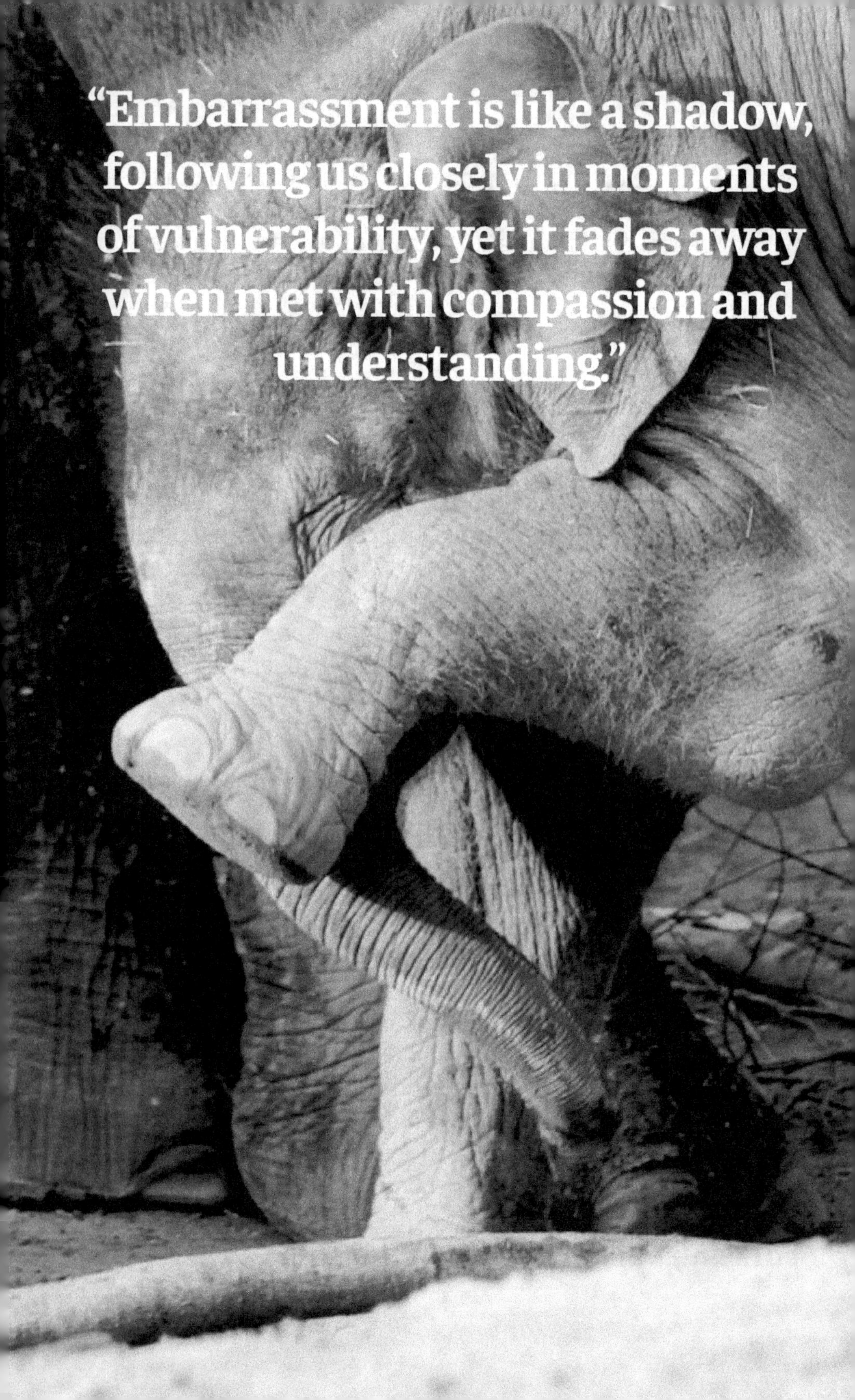

"Embarrassment is like a shadow, following us closely in moments of vulnerability, yet it fades away when met with compassion and understanding."

3.4
How It Feels for THE OTHER ONE.

Introduction

While much focus is placed on the caregiver's experience, it's equally important to acknowledge how the care recipient feels about the care they receive. For the Other One, it can be an undignified and surreal experience, profoundly impacting their mental health and well-being.

The Struggle with Loss of Dignity

For the Other One, depending on their level of awareness and cognitive function, requiring assistance with personal care tasks can be deeply humiliating. The loss of independence and the need for intimate care can strip away their sense of dignity and autonomy, leading to feelings of embarrassment, shame, and frustration.

Navigating Surreal Moments

Imagine being in the position of the Other One, where your body is no longer fully under your control, and you rely on others for basic tasks like bathing, dressing, and toileting. It can feel surreal and disorienting to suddenly find yourself in such a vulnerable position, dependent on others for your most fundamental needs.

Impact on Mental Health

The experience of receiving care can have a significant impact on the Other One's mental health. It's not uncommon for them to experience feelings of depression, anxiety, and low self-esteem as they grapple with their changed circumstances. They may feel like a burden to their caregivers, leading to feelings of guilt and worthlessness.

Maintaining Compassion and Empathy

As caregivers, it's essential to approach the care we provide with compassion, empathy, and respect for the Other One's dignity. Taking the time to listen to their concerns, preferences, and feelings can help alleviate some of the distress they may experience.

Engaging in open and honest communication, reassuring them of their worth and value, and involving them in decision-making whenever possible can help empower them and preserve their sense of dignity.

Promoting Well-being

Supporting the Other One's mental health and well-being is just as important as addressing their physical needs. Encouraging social interaction, meaningful activities, and opportunities for self-expression can help combat feelings of isolation and maintain their sense of identity and purpose.

Conclusion

While caregiving often focuses on meeting the practical needs of the care recipient, it's crucial to consider the emotional and psychological impact of receiving care. By recognizing and validating the Other One's feelings and experiences, we can provide more holistic and compassionate care that honors their dignity and preserves their well-being.

3.5
YES! You may have to do all this!

Chapter 3 has illuminated the diverse and demanding nature of caregiving, showcasing the myriad roles and responsibilities caregivers undertake. From providing personal care with dignity and empathy to navigating complex family dynamics and medical situations with diplomacy, caregivers wear many hats. The chapter emphasizes the importance of empowering care recipients while acknowledging the emotional toll and surreal experiences caregivers face.

Despite the challenges, caregivers must confront uncomfortable tasks and advocate for their loved ones' well-being. Through it all, the chapter reminds caregivers that their efforts, though often unheralded, are essential for maintaining dignity and quality of life. much focus is placed on the caregiver's experience, it's equally important to acknowledge how the care recipient feels about the care they receive. For the Other One, it can be an undignified and surreal experience, profoundly impacting their mental health and well-being.

Managing the Emotional Toll
Taking on multiple roles can be emotionally taxing. It's important to recognize the impact this has on you and take steps to manage your well-being:

- **Self-Care:** Make time for yourself, even if it's just a few minutes each day to relax and unwind.

- **Seek Support:** Connect with other caregivers through support groups or online communities to share experiences and advice.

- **Professional Help:** Consider speaking with a therapist or counsellor to manage stress and emotional challenges.

Setting Boundaries

While it's important to be supportive, setting boundaries is crucial to prevent burnout. Here are some tips for setting healthy boundaries:

- **Communicate Clearly**: Let your loved one know what you can and cannot do. Be honest about your limitations.

- **Schedule Breaks:** Plan regular breaks and respite care to ensure you have time to recharge.

- **Say No When Needed:** It's okay to say no to tasks that are beyond your capacity or that could negatively impact your well-being.

Get Your Hands Dirty!

As mentioned earlier, dive in as soon as you can. Get your hands dirty (Remember to wear gloves and PPE)

The sooner you get used to this, the better. The quicker you become a great carer!

Washing Dishes just Like Washing Me!

In the kitchen sink, a pile of dishes lay,
Awaiting their fate at the end of the day.
With soap and sponge, I roll up my sleeves,
To tackle this task and conquer with ease.

Each plate and cup tells its own little tale,
Of meals shared together, of laughter and hail.
But now they're adorned with crumbs and debris,
It's time for a scrub, for cleanliness spree!

As I lather and rinse, I ponder with glee,
Cleaning dishes is much like cleaning me.
Just like these plates, I need a good scrub,
o wash away worries and any odd flub.

The forks and knives gleam, their edges sharp,
As I cleanse away grime,
I feel a spark. For in every dish, there's a lesson to find,
About life's messes and leaving them behind.

So let's scrub away, with vigor and zest,
Embracing the task with our very best.
For cleaning dishes is more than just that,
It's a metaphor for life, imagine that!

With each gleaming dish, we're washing away,
The troubles and troubles of yesterday.
So let's suds up and rinse with glee,
For cleaning dishes is like setting us free!

CHAPTER 4

STRESS AND HOW IT AFFECTS MYSELF!

"In Alice in Wonderland, the White Rabbit's stress over being late for a very important date highlights the pressure we often place on ourselves to meet expectations and timelines. It serves as a reminder that in our hurried lives, anxiety and stress can sometimes overshadow the very moments we're rushing to experience!"

4.1
Identifying Stress and It's Sources.

Introduction

Now that we have covered in the previous chapter, what you have to do as a care givers, do you feel stressed?

Stress is an inherent part of caregiving, often lurking beneath the surface and impacting both the caregiver and the care recipient. Identifying stress and understanding its sources are crucial steps in managing its effects and maintaining mental well-being. In this module, we will explore what stress is, its common sources in the caregiving context, and how it can manifest in daily life.

Understanding Stress.

Stress is the body's response to any demand or challenge that disrupts our normal balance. It triggers a cascade of physical, emotional, and behavioural reactions designed to help us cope with perceived threats. While a certain level of stress can be motivating and even beneficial, chronic stress can have detrimental effects on our health and well-being. For caregivers, stress often becomes a constant companion, driven by the myriad responsibilities and emotional demands of caregiving.

Common Sources of Stress in Caregiving

- **Physical Demands** Caregiving is physically demanding work. From lifting and moving a loved one to managing household chores and medical tasks, the physical toll can be immense. These physical demands can lead to fatigue, muscle strain, and even injuries, contributing significantly to caregiver stress.

- **Emotional Strain** The emotional strain of caregiving cannot be overstated. Witnessing the decline of a loved one, dealing with their mood swings, and managing the psychological impact of their condition can be overwhelming. The constant emotional rollercoaster, coupled with feelings of helplessness and frustration, can intensify stress levels.

- **Time Pressure Time** management is a perpetual challenge for caregivers. Balancing caregiving responsibilities with personal and professional obligations often leaves little room for self-care. The relentless pressure to be constantly available can lead to a sense of being perpetually rushed and overwhelmed.

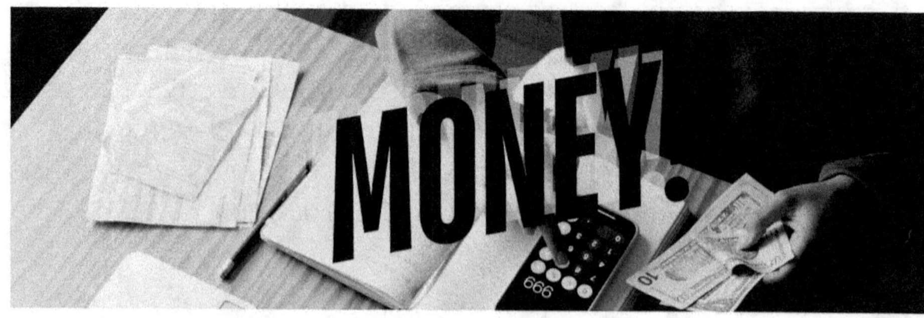

- **Financial Concerns** Financial stress is a common concern among caregivers. The costs associated with medical care, medications, and necessary home modifications can quickly add up. For many, the financial burden is compounded by the need to reduce working hours or leave employment entirely, leading to increased anxiety and stress.

- **Social Isolation** Caregiving can be an isolating experience. The demands of caregiving often leave little time for social interactions, leading to feelings of loneliness and isolation. The lack of social support can exacerbate stress, making it harder to cope with the daily challenges of caregiving.

- **Uncertainty and Lack of Control** The unpredictable nature of many health conditions can create a sense of uncertainty and lack of control. Caregivers may feel anxious about the future and overwhelmed by the unpredictability of their loved one's condition. This uncertainty can be a significant source of stress.

- **Fear of the Unknown and Understanding the Condition** Fear of the unknown is a pervasive stressor in caregiving. Understanding the condition your loved one is experiencing and anticipating its progression can be daunting. The lack of clear information and the unpredictability of symptoms can create an ongoing sense of fear and anxiety. Caregivers may struggle to comprehend complex medical information, feel unsure about how to respond to changes, and worry about what the future holds. This fear can be compounded by the emotional burden of seeing a loved one suffer and feeling powerless to help.

Manifestations of Stress in Caregivers

- **Physical Symptoms** Stress often manifests physically. Common symptoms include headaches, muscle tension, fatigue, sleep disturbances, and gastrointestinal issues. Chronic stress can weaken the immune system, making caregivers more susceptible to illnesses.

- **Emotional and Psychological Symptoms** Emotionally, stress can lead to feelings of anxiety, depression, irritability, and mood swings. Caregivers may experience a sense of dread or panic, struggle with concentration and decision-making, and feel persistently overwhelmed or helpless.

- **Behavioural Changes** Behavioural changes are another indicator of stress. These might include withdrawing from social activities, neglecting personal care, changes in eating habits, increased use of alcohol or other substances, and a decline in productivity or performance at work.

Example:

Identifying Stress in a Caregiver Consider Jane, who has been caring for her husband, Tom, who has advanced Parkinson's disease. Jane's daily routine is filled with tasks: administering medication, assisting with mobility, and managing household chores. Over time, Jane begins to experience chronic headaches, fatigue, and insomnia. Emotionally, she feels increasingly irritable and overwhelmed, often finding herself in tears. She starts to withdraw from friends and neglects her hobbies. Recognizing these signs, Jane acknowledges that stress is taking a toll on her well-being and decides to seek support and strategies to manage her stress.

Conclusion

Identifying stress and its sources is the first step in managing its impact. By understanding the common sources of stress in caregiving and recognizing its manifestations, caregivers can take proactive steps to address their stress and maintain their well-being. In the next module, we will explore strategies for managing stress, providing practical tools and techniques to help caregivers navigate their challenging roles with resilience and strength.

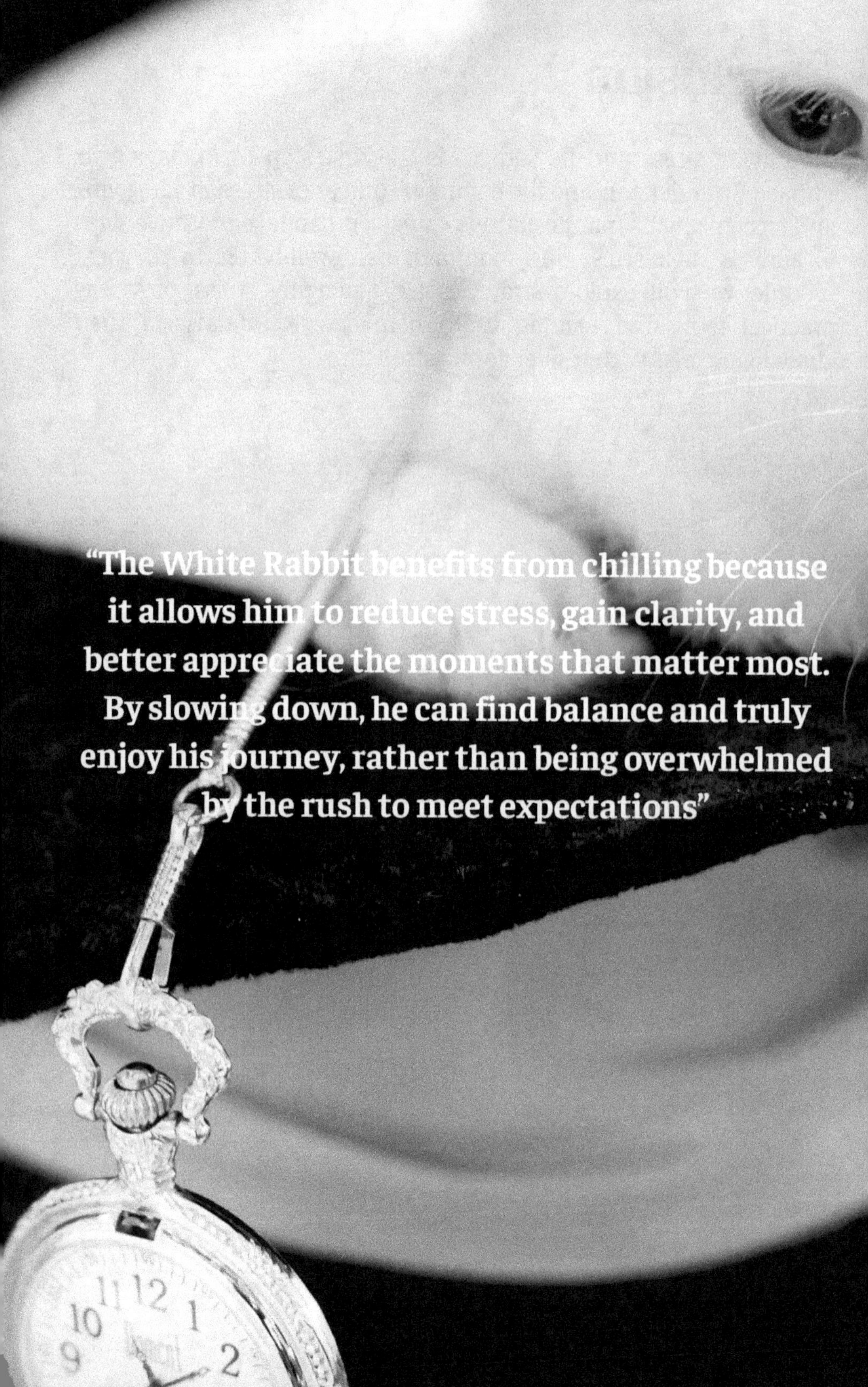

"The White Rabbit benefits from chilling because it allows him to reduce stress, gain clarity, and better appreciate the moments that matter most. By slowing down, he can find balance and truly enjoy his journey, rather than being overwhelmed by the rush to meet expectations"

4.2
Stress and Trauma with THE OTHER ONE and How It Affects MYSELF

Introduction

Caregiving can be an emotionally intense experience, often intertwined with moments of trauma. This module will explore the concept of stress and trauma within caregiving, identifying both fast and slow triggers, and how these experiences impact both caregivers and care recipients. Understanding these elements is crucial for developing resilience and effective coping strategies.

Understanding Stress and Trauma

Stress and trauma in caregiving are often interlinked. Trauma can result from witnessing a loved one's suffering, dealing with their unpredictable behaviors, or experiencing a critical incident. This trauma can lead to chronic stress, affecting the caregiver's mental health and overall well-being. Recognizing the signs of trauma and understanding its triggers is essential for mitigating its impact.

One source of stress, as discussed in the previous chapter, is the volume of tasks caregivers must manage. From scheduling medical appointments to administering medications, and providing emotional support to performing household chores, the demands are endless. This constant juggling act, without adequate breaks or assistance, can create a high-pressure environment where stress and trauma thrive.

Trauma in caregiving isn't always about major incidents; it can also stem from cumulative stress. For instance, dealing with a loved one's erratic behavior due to dementia or chronic illness can be emotionally draining. Each unpredictable episode chips away at the caregiver's resilience, gradually leading to chronic stress.

Fast Triggers

Immediate Reactions
Fast triggers are immediate, sudden events that provoke a quick and intense stress response, much like a cowboy shootout. These rapid-fire situations leave no time to think, only to react.

Partner and Shouting: Imagine a scenario where your partner suddenly starts shouting during a disagreement. This can feel like a gunfight at high noon, causing an instant spike in stress, marked by a rapid heartbeat, sweating, and a rush of adrenaline.

Care Situations: In caregiving, fast triggers can occur when a loved one has a sudden fall, a medical emergency, or an unexpected outburst. For instance, if you're assisting a loved one with dementia who suddenly becomes agitated and aggressive, it can feel like a surprise ambush, provoking a swift and intense stress response.

Impact on Caregiving
Fast triggers in caregiving often demand immediate action, leaving little time to process emotions. These situations can lead to heightened anxiety, increased irritability, and a feeling of being constantly on edge. It's akin to living in a perpetual state of high alert, ready to react at a moment's notice, which can severely impact a caregiver's mental and emotional well-being.

Here's a quote inspired by John Wayne about two gunfighters in a shootout. The same can be said about fast triggers.

"In a shootout, it's not about who draws first, but who stays calm and aims true. Two gunfighters face off, but it's the one with steady nerves who walks away."

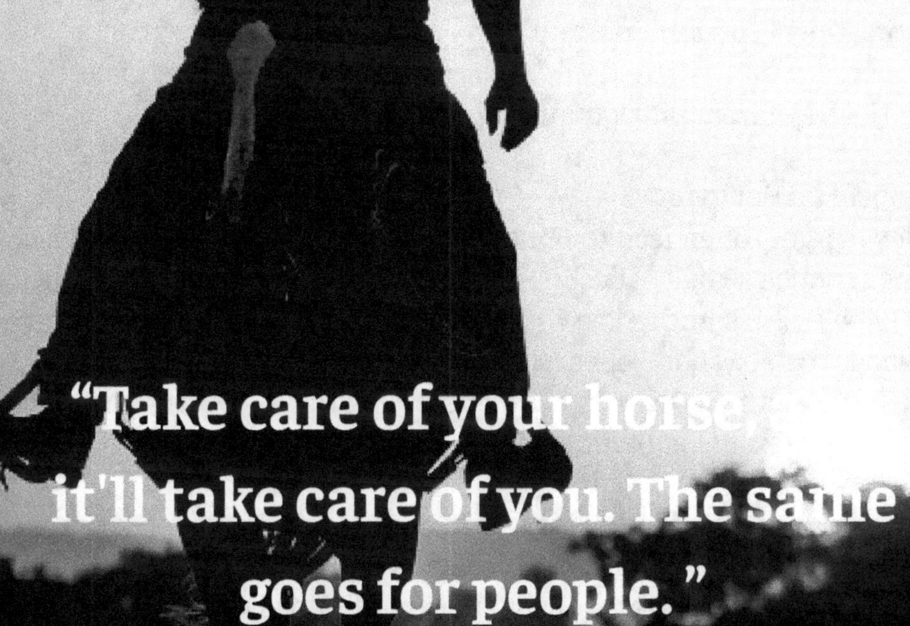

This quote captures the cowboy spirit of mutual care and respect, emphasizing that the well-being of others, whether animals or people, directly impacts one's own well-being.

3. Slow Triggers

What is your routine in the morning? Do you get up, use the bathroom, have a coffee, and listen to the news? What happens when your routine is broken? It can throw your entire day off balance. This disruption could be the first of many slow triggers that gradually build up, leading to chronic stress. How about the person you support. How does this affect them? Slow triggers are more insidious, accumulating over time and leading to chronic stress. Here are some examples:

Long-Term Care Responsibilities: The gradual accumulation of caregiving tasks without adequate breaks or support can be a slow trigger. The constant physical and emotional demands can slowly build up, leading to burnout.

Persistent Worries: Constant worry about your loved one's condition, finances, or future care needs can act as a slow trigger. Over time, this can lead to chronic anxiety and depression.

Impact on Behavior

Slow triggers often lead to underlying behavioral changes. Caregivers might notice a gradual decline in their enthusiasm, increased feelings of hopelessness, and a slow withdrawal from social interactions. These changes can be subtle but accumulate to have a significant impact on mental health. Recognizing and addressing these slow triggers early can help prevent long-term emotional and psychological harm.

Slow triggers are like boiling a kettle. Initially, the water heats up slowly, with little visible change. However, as the heat continues to build, the temperature gradually rises until it finally reaches a boiling point, causing the kettle to whistle. Similarly, slow triggers in caregiving accumulate over time, each small stressor adding to the next. Eventually, without adequate breaks or support, these stressors can build up to a critical point, leading to a sudden onset of burnout or a significant decline in mental health. Recognizing and managing these slow triggers early can help prevent reaching that boiling point.

The Impact of Trauma

Psychological Effects
Trauma can leave lasting psychological scars. Caregivers may experience symptoms of post-traumatic stress disorder (PTSD), including flashbacks, nightmares, and severe anxiety. The trauma of witnessing a loved one's suffering or dealing with their unpredictable behaviors can lead to long-term emotional distress.

Trauma in those you support can be deep-rooted, often stemming from past incidents. This deep-seated trauma frequently causes individuals to rely on their emotional brain rather than their thinking brain, leading to more frequent and intense triggers. When caregivers use their emotional brain, it not only stresses "The Other One" (the person they are caring for) but also affects "Me" (the caregiver).

Behavioral Manifestations
Trauma can also manifest in various behaviors, often linked to past experiences:

Hypervigilance: Caregivers may become overly alert and anxious, constantly on the lookout for potential crises.

Avoidance: Some may start avoiding situations or tasks that remind them of traumatic experiences, leading to the neglect of important caregiving duties.

Emotional Numbing: To cope with trauma, caregivers might emotionally detach, becoming less responsive or compassionate over time.

Example: Recognizing Trauma in a Caregiver Consider Mark, who cares for his mother with Alzheimer's disease. Over time, he has witnessed her decline and experienced numerous distressing incidents, such as her wandering off and getting lost. These experiences have left Mark hypervigilant, constantly anxious about her safety. He finds himself avoiding taking her out for walks, fearing she might get lost again.

Additionally, Mark has become emotionally numb, feeling detached from both his mother and his own family. Recognizing these signs of trauma, Mark seeks professional help to address his symptoms and improve his caregiving approach.

Conclusion

Understanding the interplay between stress and trauma in caregiving is essential for maintaining both your well-being and that of your loved one. By identifying fast and slow triggers and recognizing the impact of trauma, caregivers can take proactive steps to address these challenges. In the next module, we will explore strategies for managing stress and trauma, equipping you with the tools to navigate the caregiving journey with resilience and strength.

Avoid
the
avoidable

4.3
Physical and Emotional Effects of Stress

Stress is an inevitable part of caregiving, with significant emotional and physical demands. While some stress can be manageable, chronic stress profoundly impacts caregivers' mental and physical health. Understanding these effects is crucial for maintaining well-being and providing quality care. This module explores the physical and emotional effects of stress, its impact on mental health, and how behavior breeds behavior, creating a cycle of mirrored stress between caregivers and care recipients.

Physical Effects of Stress

Fatigue and Sleep Disturbances Chronic stress often leads to fatigue and sleep disturbances, as caregiving demands make rest difficult. Lack of sleep exacerbates stress, depleting the caregiver's energy and reducing their ability to provide effective care.

Headaches and Muscle Stress triggers the release of hormones like cortisol, causing headaches and muscle tension. Caregivers may experience migraines and tightness in the neck, shoulders, and back, further diminishing their ability to manage tasks.

Gastrointestinal Problems The gastrointestinal system is highly sensitive to stress. Chronic stress can lead to a range of digestive issues, including stomach aches, constipation, diarrhoea, and irritable bowel syndrome (IBS). These symptoms can be particularly disruptive, affecting the caregiver's daily functioning and overall quality of life.

Cardiovascular Issues Prolonged stress is a significant risk factor for cardiovascular problems. Caregivers under constant stress may experience high blood pressure, increased heart rate, and a higher risk of heart disease and stroke. The strain on the cardiovascular system can be life-threatening if not managed properly.

Weakened Immune System Stress weakens the immune system, making caregivers more susceptible to infections and illnesses. Frequent colds, flu, and other infections can become common, further straining the caregiver's ability to fulfil their responsibilities and maintain their health.

Example: *Physical Effects on a Caregiver Consider Sarah, who has been caring for her father with Alzheimer's disease. Over time, Sarah begins to experience chronic fatigue and frequent tension headaches. She also notices that she's getting colds more often and has developed stomach aches that disrupt her daily routine. These physical symptoms, exacerbated by the relentless demands of caregiving, highlight the toll that chronic stress can take on a caregiver's body.*

Emotional Effects of Stress

Anxiety and Depression Chronic stress is a major contributor to anxiety and depression. The constant pressure and emotional demands of caregiving can lead to feelings of worry, hopelessness, and sadness. Caregivers may experience panic attacks, excessive worry about their loved one's health, and a pervasive sense of dread about the future.

Irritability and Mood Swings Stress can cause significant emotional instability. Caregivers under chronic stress may find themselves easily irritated, prone to mood swings, and quick to anger. This emotional volatility can strain relationships with the care recipient and other family members, leading to further emotional distress.

Feelings of Guilt and Inadequacy Many caregivers struggle with feelings of guilt and inadequacy. They may feel that they are not doing enough for their loved one, or that they are failing in their caregiving duties. This sense of guilt can be overwhelming, leading to a decline in self-esteem and further contributing to emotional stress.

Emotional Numbing To cope with the constant emotional strain, some caregivers may become emotionally numb, detaching themselves from their feelings as a protective mechanism. This emotional detachment can lead to a loss of joy in activities they once enjoyed and a disconnection from loved ones, compounding their sense of isolation.

Example: *Emotional Effects on a Caregiver Take John, who cares for his wife with advanced multiple sclerosis. John finds himself increasingly anxious, worrying about his wife's condition and the future. He becomes easily irritated and often snaps at his children, causing tension within the family. Over time, John starts to feel numb, unable to find joy in his hobbies or interactions with friends, leading to a deeper sense of isolation and despair.*

Behavioural Effects of Stress

Changes in Eating Habits Stress often leads to changes in eating habits, which can be detrimental to health. Some caregivers may eat more than usual, turning to comfort foods that are high in sugar and fat. Others may lose their appetite altogether, leading to poor nutrition and weight loss.

Increased Use of Substances To cope with stress, some caregivers may turn to substances such as alcohol, tobacco, or drugs. While these might provide temporary relief, they ultimately exacerbate stress and lead to further health problems, creating a destructive cycle that is hard to break.

Social Withdrawal Chronic stress can lead caregivers to withdraw from social activities and isolate themselves. The demands of caregiving often leave little time or energy for social interactions, and caregivers may feel too overwhelmed or depressed to engage with friends and family. This isolation further compounds their stress and emotional distress.

Neglect of Personal Care Caregivers under chronic stress may neglect their own personal care. This can include skipping medical appointments, not exercising, and neglecting basic hygiene. The constant focus on the needs of the care recipient can lead to caregivers overlooking their own health and well-being.

Example: *Behavioural Effects on a Caregiver Imagine Linda, who takes care of her son with severe autism. Under constant stress, Linda starts eating irregularly, skipping meals, and relying on fast food. She begins to drink wine every evening to unwind, which gradually becomes a daily habit. Linda also withdraws from her social circle, feeling too exhausted to meet friends or participate in community events. As she becomes more isolated, her stress levels rise, creating a cycle that further impacts her health and ability to care for her son.*

Behaviour Breeds Behaviour: Mirroring Stress

The Cycle of Mirrored Stress Behaviour breeds behaviour, meaning that stress in caregivers can be mirrored by the care recipients, creating a cycle of stress that affects both parties. When caregivers are stressed, their loved ones often pick up on these emotional cues, leading to increased anxiety and stress in the care recipient. This reciprocal stress can exacerbate existing conditions and create a more challenging caregiving environment.

Examples of Mirrored Stress

Partner and Shouting: In a household where arguments and shouting are common due to stress, both the caregiver and the care recipient can become more anxious and irritable. For instance, if a caregiver shouts at their partner out of frustration, the partner may become more agitated and uncooperative, escalating the situation further.

Care Situations: In caregiving, if a caregiver is visibly stressed and anxious, the care recipient might mirror these emotions. For example, a caregiver's tense body language and hurried movements can make a person with dementia feel anxious and confused, leading to increased agitation and behavioural issues.

Slow Triggers and Underlying Behaviours

Slow triggers are more insidious and can lead to underlying behaviours that reflect accumulated stress. These can include:

Resentment Building: Over time, the slow build-up of caregiving responsibilities without respite can lead to feelings of resentment. This resentment may manifest in passive-aggressive behaviour or a lack of patience with the care recipient.

Chronic Worry: Persistent worry about the care recipient's health or future can lead to a constant state of stress, affecting the caregiver's interactions and decisions. This chronic worry can manifest in overprotective or controlling behaviours, further stressing the care recipient.

Example: *Mirroring Stress in Caregiving Consider Mike, who cares for his elderly mother with dementia. Mike's chronic stress leads to irritability and a short temper. When he becomes frustrated, he often raises his voice, causing his mother to become more agitated and confused. This reaction increases Mike's stress, creating a vicious cycle. Additionally, Mike's slow-building resentment about the lack of support leads him to withdraw emotionally, which his mother senses, causing her to feel more isolated and anxious.*

Impact of Trauma

Psychological Effects of Trauma Caregiving can sometimes involve traumatic experiences, such as witnessing a loved one's severe decline or dealing with medical emergencies. Trauma can have lasting psychological effects, including symptoms of post-traumatic stress disorder (PTSD) like flashbacks, nightmares, and severe anxiety. These traumatic experiences can deeply affect the caregiver's mental health and ability to provide care.

Behavioural Manifestations of Trauma Trauma can also manifest in behaviours that are influenced by past experiences. These behaviours can include:

Hypervigilance: Caregivers may become excessively alert and anxious, always anticipating the next crisis. This hypervigilance can lead to burnout and emotional exhaustion.

Avoidance: Some caregivers might avoid certain tasks or situations that remind them of traumatic events, leading to neglect of essential caregiving duties.

Emotional Numbing: To cope with trauma, caregivers might emotionally detach, leading to a lack of responsiveness and compassion, which can impact the quality of care provided.

Example: *Trauma in a Caregiver Consider Emily, who witnessed her father's traumatic stroke. The experience left her with severe anxiety and frequent flashbacks. Emily becomes hypervigilant, constantly checking her father's vital signs and overreacting to minor health changes. She also avoids certain caregiving tasks that remind her of the stroke, leading to gaps in his care. This trauma-induced behaviour affects both her well-being and her father's care.*

Conclusion

The physical and emotional effects of stress in caregiving are profound and multifaceted. By understanding these effects and recognizing the signs of stress and trauma, caregivers can take steps to address their well-being. Recognizing that behaviour breeds behaviour is crucial in breaking the cycle of mirrored stress between caregivers and care recipients. In the next module, we will explore strategies for managing stress and trauma, providing practical tools to navigate the caregiving journey with resilience and strength.

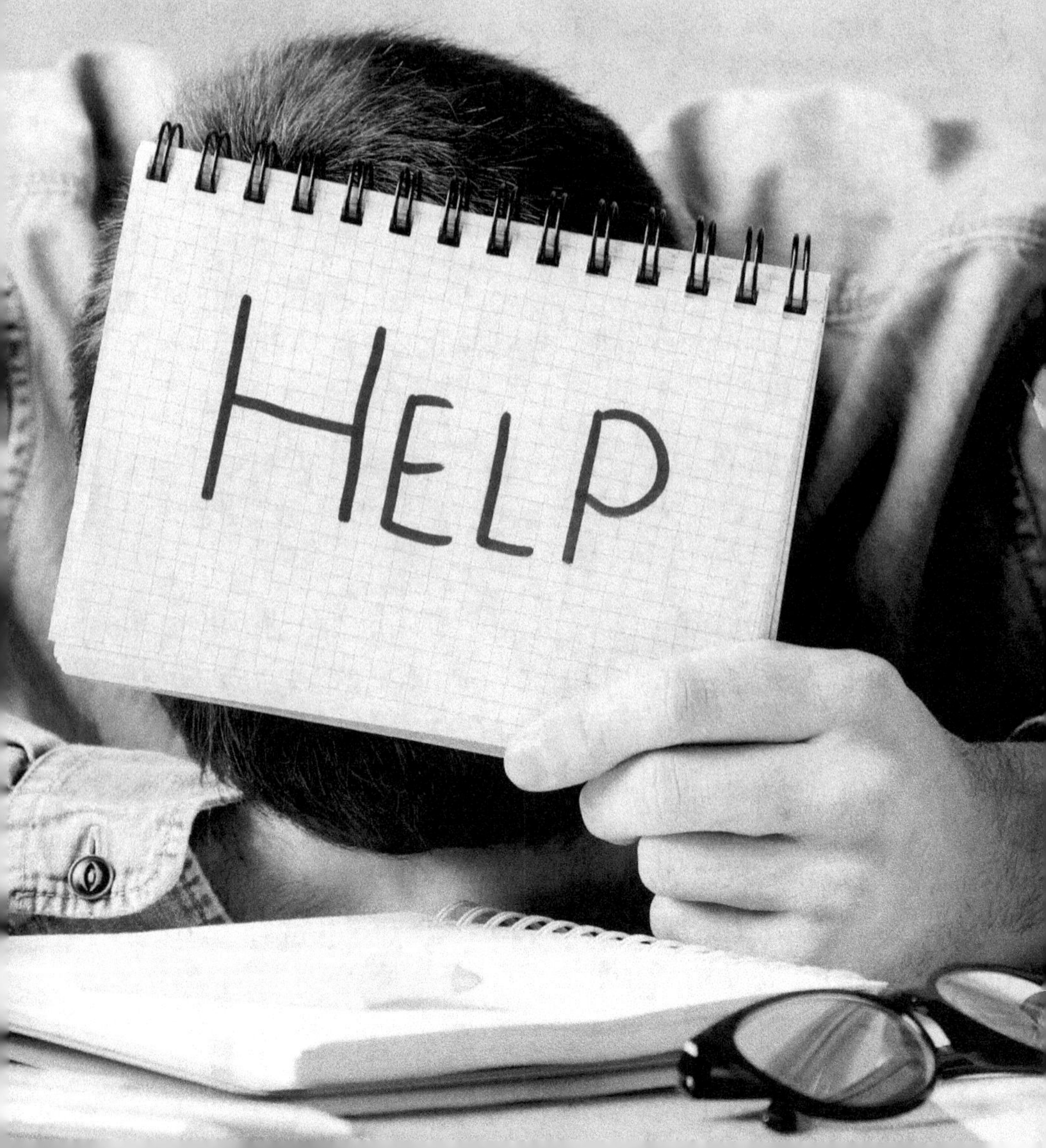

4.4
Don't Let It Get to You- Think of MYSELF

Stress and trauma are formidable challenges in the caregiving journey, but it's crucial to remember that you have the power to manage and mitigate their impact. It might feel overwhelming at times, but with the right mindset and tools, you can maintain your well-being and provide the best care for your loved one.

You Are Not Alone Many caregivers face similar struggles, and it's important to recognize that you are not alone in this. Sharing experiences and connecting with others can provide much-needed support and perspective. Understanding that these feelings are a common part of the caregiving experience can be reassuring.

The Power of Resilience Resilience is the ability to bounce back from adversity, and it can be cultivated. By building resilience, you can navigate the ups and downs of caregiving with greater ease and confidence. This book will offer strategies to help you develop resilience and cope with stress effectively.

Look Forward to Practical Strategies In the upcoming chapters, we will delve into practical strategies and techniques to help you manage stress, address trauma, and improve your overall well-being. From mindfulness exercises to time management tips, you will find tools that are both easy to implement and effective.

Conclusion

Don't let stress and trauma define your caregiving experience. By staying proactive and open to new approaches, you can create a more manageable and positive caregiving journey. Stay tuned for the next modules, where we will explore actionable strategies to support your mental health and enhance your caregiving role.

The Greek Gods Also Got Stressed

On Olympus, the gods felt distressed,
Caring for mortals left them quite stressed.
Zeus sighed with a thunderous boom,
While Hera just tidied her room.

Apollo played tunes that were blue,
Artemis wondered what to do.
Athena's wisdom felt quite thin,
Ares just wanted to win.

Poseidon's waves crashed in despair,
Aphrodite's hair lost its flair.
Hephaestus's forge lacked its spark,
Demeter's crops stayed in the dark.

Hermes ran errands with a groan,
Dionysus drank wine all alone.
Even Hades peeked from the gloom,
To see if the stress would consume.

So they all took a godly retreat,
To a spa that was truly elite.
With massages divine,
And ambrosia wine,
They found bliss in their heavenly suite.

"Let's leave mortals to their own quest,"
Said Zeus, feeling much more at rest.
The gods all agreed,
They had earned this indeed,
Caring's tough, even for the blessed!

CHAPTER 5

UNDERSTANDING ANXIETY AND DEPRESSION!

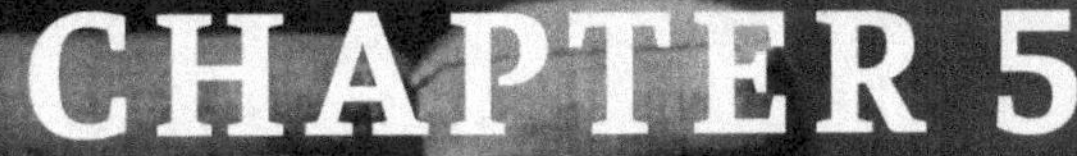

"Staying positive serves as a crucial sanity check, helping to overcome depression and anxiety by fostering resilience and providing a hopeful perspective in challenging times!"

5.1
Understanding Anxiety and Depression.

Introduction

Caregiving is an immensely demanding and often exhausting role that can take a significant toll on one's mental health. Among the most common mental health challenges caregivers face are anxiety and depression. These conditions can severely impact a caregiver's ability to provide effective care and can also negatively affect their own quality of life. In this module, we will explore what anxiety and depression are, how they manifest in caregivers, and why it is crucial to address these conditions proactively.

What Are Anxiety and Depression?

Anxiety is a feeling of worry, nervousness, or unease about something with an uncertain outcome. While it is a normal reaction to stress, chronic anxiety is characterized by persistent and excessive worry that interferes with daily activities. Common symptoms include restlessness, rapid heartbeat, difficulty concentrating, and muscle tension. According to the Anxiety and Depression Association of America (ADAA), anxiety disorders affect 40 million adults in the United States every year. In the UK, anxiety disorders are estimated to affect around 8.2 million people.

Depression, on the other hand, is a mood disorder that causes a persistent feeling of sadness and loss of interest. It affects how you feel, think, and handle daily activities. Symptoms include feelings of hopelessness, lack of energy, changes in appetite or sleep patterns, and difficulty concentrating. In severe cases, depression can lead to thoughts of suicide. The National Institute of Mental Health (NIMH) reports that approximately 17.3 million adults in the U.S. experienced at least one major depressive episode in 2017. In England, around 3.3 million people are diagnosed with depression each year.

The Link Between Caregiving, Anxiety, and Depression

Caregivers are particularly vulnerable to anxiety and depression due to the constant demands and pressures associated with their role. The responsibility of caring for a loved one, often combined with other personal and professional obligations, can lead to significant emotional and physical stress. This chronic stress can trigger or exacerbate anxiety and depression. Studies have shown that up to 70% of caregivers exhibit clinically significant symptoms of depression, with approximately one in five meeting the diagnostic criteria for major depression. In the UK, around 40% of caregivers report experiencing depression.

The Unique Stressors of Caregiving

Several unique stressors contribute to anxiety and depression among caregivers:

Emotional Strain: Witnessing a loved one's decline can be heart breaking and emotionally draining. The sadness and grief associated with watching someone you care about suffer can lead to feelings of hopelessness and despair. This emotional burden is compounded by the need to maintain a strong and supportive presence for the care recipient.

Isolation: Caregivers often find themselves isolated, as their responsibilities can limit their ability to maintain social connections. This isolation can lead to loneliness, which is a significant risk factor for depression. According to a study by AARP, 46% of caregivers report feeling isolated, which exacerbates their emotional distress. In the UK, around 57% of caregivers feel socially isolated as a result of their caregiving responsibilities.

Lack of Support: Many caregivers do not have adequate support from family, friends, or professional services. This lack of support can make caregivers feel overwhelmed and alone, exacerbating feelings of anxiety and depression. In a survey by the NAC, 36% of caregivers reported that their caregiving situation was highly stressful, partly due to the lack of adequate support. Similarly, in England, about one-third of caregiver's report feeling unsupported in their role.

Financial Pressure: The financial burden of caregiving can be substantial, especially if it involves paying for medical treatments, medications, and other care-related expenses. Financial stress is a common trigger for anxiety and depression. The National Alliance for Caregiving (NAC) found that nearly half of caregivers spend more than $5,000 annually on out-of-pocket caregiving costs. In the UK, the Carers Trust estimates that caregivers save the economy around £132 billion annually, yet many face significant financial hardships themselves.

Doing unfamiliar Things: Many first time care givers worry about the tasks they have to perform. These could include personal care, manual handling people, giving medication or even communicating the OTHER ONES's needs to people. Sometimes this can affect people.

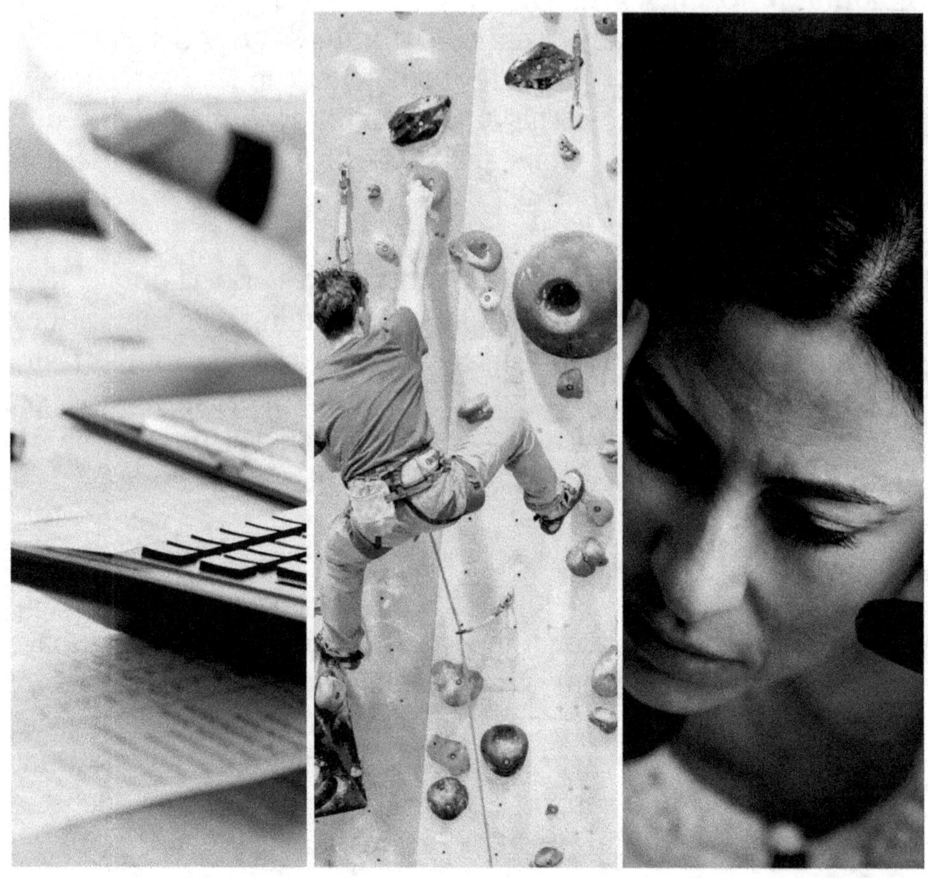

EMILY'S STORY

Emily has been caring for her husband, who has Parkinson's disease, for the past five years. Initially, she managed well, balancing caregiving with her part-time job and social activities. However, as her husband's condition worsened, Emily's responsibilities increased. She started experiencing constant worry about his health and future, which led to sleepless nights and physical symptoms like headaches and muscle tension. Eventually, Emily began to feel overwhelmed and hopeless, losing interest in activities she once enjoyed. Her friends noticed that she had become withdrawn and irritable. Emily's persistent sadness and feelings of worthlessness were classic signs of depression, compounded by anxiety about her husband's care.

5.2
Mirror Mirror: How Anxiety and Depression Affect Those You Support and Vice Versa

Caregiving is a deeply interconnected experience. The emotional and mental states of both the caregiver and the person being cared for are intricately linked, often influencing each other in profound ways. Anxiety and depression can create a feedback loop where the mental health of one person affects the other, leading to a cycle of mirrored behaviours and emotions. This module will explore how anxiety and depression can affect both caregivers and care recipients, highlighting the ways in which behaviours are mirrored and the impact this can have on the caregiving dynamic.

The Emotional Echo: How Behaviours are Mirrored

Human beings are naturally empathetic creatures, and this empathy can lead to the mirroring of emotions and behaviours. When a caregiver feels anxious or depressed, these emotions can subtly influence their interactions with the care recipient. Similarly, the emotional state of the person being cared for can affect the caregiver. This phenomenon is known as emotional contagion, where one person's emotions and related behaviours trigger similar emotions and behaviours in another person.

Examples of Mirrored Behaviours

Monotone Speech and Mood Matching:

If a caregiver is feeling depressed, they may speak in a monotone voice, lacking enthusiasm or warmth. The person being cared for can pick up on these cues, leading to a decrease in their own mood and responsiveness. This can create a feedback loop where the caregiver perceives the care recipient's subdued mood as a lack of engagement, further deepening their own depression.

Isolation and Withdrawal:

A caregiver experiencing depression may withdraw socially, reducing interactions and activities. The care recipient, mirroring this behaviour, might also become more withdrawn, leading to increased feelings of loneliness and isolation for both parties. This mutual withdrawal can exacerbate depressive symptoms on both sides.

Case Study: Tom and His Mother, Jean

Tom has been caring for his mother, Jean, who has Alzheimer's disease, for three years. Over time, Tom's anxiety about Jean's worsening condition grew, and he began to feel overwhelmed. His anxious behaviours—such as checking on Jean frequently, pacing, and speaking in a hurried manner—started to impact Jean, who began to show signs of increased agitation and confusion. As Jean's distress grew, she became more difficult to manage, which in turn heightened Tom's anxiety. This cycle of mirrored anxiety led to a tense and stressful caregiving environment.

The Impact on Care Recipients

The mental health of caregivers plays a crucial role in the well-being of care recipients. When caregivers are anxious or depressed, it can lead to:

Increased Stress for Care Recipients

Care recipients are sensitive to the emotional states of their caregivers. If the caregiver is stressed, the care recipient is likely to experience increased stress, which can worsen their own mental and physical health condition.

Reduced Quality of Care

Depression and anxiety can impair a caregiver's ability to provide attentive and compassionate care. This can lead to a decline in the quality of care, negatively affecting the health and happiness of the care recipient.

Emotional Disconnect

When a caregiver is emotionally distressed, they may find it challenging to connect on an emotional level with the care recipient. This disconnect can lead to feelings of neglect and loneliness for the person being cared for.

The Impact on Caregivers

Conversely, the mental health of care recipients can also have a profound impact on caregivers:

Increased Caregiving Burden

If the care recipient is experiencing heightened anxiety or depression, they may require more attention and support, increasing the caregiver's burden. This added stress can worsen the caregiver's own mental health.

Emotional Drain

Witnessing a loved one suffer from anxiety or depression can be emotionally draining for caregivers. The constant exposure to negative emotions can lead to compassion fatigue, where the caregiver becomes emotionally exhausted and less able to provide care.

Feelings of Helplessness

Caregivers may feel helpless when they see their efforts to provide comfort and care are not alleviating the care recipient's distress. This sense of helplessness can contribute to the caregiver's own feelings of anxiety and depression.

Understanding the Cycle

It is crucial to recognize and understand the cycle of mirrored behaviours and emotions in caregiving. Awareness of this cycle can help caregivers identify when their own mental health might be affecting their care recipient and vice versa. By recognizing these patterns, caregivers can take proactive steps to break the cycle and create a healthier emotional environment for both themselves and their loved ones.

Conclusion

The emotional and mental health of caregivers and care recipients are closely intertwined. Anxiety and depression can create a feedback loop of mirrored behaviours and emotions, impacting both parties. Understanding this dynamic is essential for breaking the cycle and fostering a more positive caregiving environment. In the upcoming modules, we will explore strategies for managing anxiety and depression, helping caregivers and care recipients support each other in maintaining mental well-being. Remember, it is possible to create a balanced and nurturing caregiving relationship where both parties can thrive.

5.3
Symptoms and Diagnosis

Recognizing the symptoms of anxiety and depression is the first step toward getting the help you need. Both caregivers and care recipients are susceptible to these mental health challenges, and understanding the signs can lead to timely and effective intervention. This module will outline common symptoms of anxiety and depression and guide you on how to seek a proper diagnosis.

Symptoms of Anxiety

Anxiety can manifest in various ways, impacting both the mind and body. Ask yourself the following questions to determine if you might be experiencing anxiety:

Persistent Worry: Are you constantly worried about your caregiving duties or your loved one's health?

Physical Symptoms: Do you experience a rapid heartbeat, sweating, trembling, or shortness of breath?

Restlessness: Do you find it hard to relax or sit still?

Sleep Disturbances: Are you having trouble falling or staying asleep because of worry?

Concentration Issues: Is it difficult for you to focus on tasks or make decisions?

If you answered "yes" to several of these questions, you might be experiencing anxiety. It's important to recognize that anxiety can vary in intensity and can be influenced by the daily stressors of caregiving.

Symptoms of Depression

Depression often presents with a range of emotional and physical symptoms. Reflect on the following questions to assess whether you might be dealing with depression:

Persistent Sadness: Have you felt sad, empty, or hopeless most of the time for more than two weeks?

Loss of Interest: Have you lost interest in activities you once enjoyed, such as hobbies or socializing?

Fatigue: Do you feel tired all the time, even after a good night's sleep?

Changes in Appetite: Have you noticed significant changes in your eating habits or weight?

Sleep Issues: Are you sleeping too much or too little?

Feelings of Worthlessness: Do you feel excessively guilty or have low self-esteem?

Concentration Problems: Is it hard for you to concentrate, make decisions, or remember things?

Physical Aches and Pains: Do you experience unexplained aches, pains, or digestive issues?

Thoughts of Death or Suicide: Have you had thoughts about death or suicide, even if you would not act on them?

If you recognize several of these symptoms in yourself or your care recipient, it is important to seek professional help.

A PERSONAL EVENT

A few years back, I unexpectedly found myself unemployed. Alongside this, I was grappling with several personal and financial problems that seemed to pile up relentlessly. I didn't realize the extent to which all these issues had affected me until one morning when I decided to take a drive. It was early, and I felt an overwhelming need to get out of the house, away from my thoughts and the suffocating atmosphere.

As I drove, the quiet of the morning seemed to offer a brief respite. However, on the way back home, my mind wandered to the multitude of problems I was facing. Without even realizing it, I had driven almost 20 miles in the opposite direction. The realization hit me hard—I wasn't just lost on the road but in life. This was more than a momentary lapse; it was a clear indication that I was deeply depressed. I realised that this must have been triggered by what I had been thinking the night before. With a the company of a bottle of whiskey in one hand, I had been thinking the unthinkable.

But that changed after this drive. I started to rethink things.

In the weeks following this incident, I stumbled upon the world of caregiving. At first, it was just a job to fill the time and pay the bills, but it quickly became much more. I found a sense of purpose in caring for others, a way to channel my energy positively and constructively.

Each day, I made it a point to find something positive, something that brought a smile to my face or someone else's. Caring for others gave me a new lease on life.

I no longer dwell on the past or my problems but instead focused on making each day a positive experience. Since then, I haven't looked back. Every day, I embrace the opportunity to make a difference, turning what was once a dark period into a journey of growth and fulfillment.

5.4
Symptoms and Diagnosis

Seeking a Diagnosis

Identifying symptoms is only the first step. A proper diagnosis from a healthcare professional is crucial for effective treatment. Here's what you can do:

Schedule an Appointment: Make an appointment with your primary care doctor or a mental health specialist. They can conduct a thorough evaluation and refer you to a psychologist or psychiatrist if necessary.

Be Honest and Open: During your appointment, be honest about what you're experiencing. Describe your symptoms in detail, including their frequency and intensity.

Complete Assessments: Your healthcare provider may ask you to complete questionnaires or assessments to better understand your mental health.

Discuss Your Role as a Caregiver: Explain your caregiving responsibilities. This context is essential for understanding the sources of your anxiety and depression.

Example: John's Experience

John, a caregiver for his elderly father with Parkinson's disease, began noticing he was frequently irritable, had trouble sleeping, and felt a persistent sense of dread. At first, he attributed these feelings to the stress of caregiving. However, after reading about the symptoms of anxiety and depression, he realized he needed professional help. John scheduled an appointment with his doctor, who diagnosed him with anxiety and depression. With a treatment plan that included therapy and medication, John gradually began to manage his symptoms better and felt more equipped to handle his caregiving responsibilities.

Conclusion

Understanding and recognizing the symptoms of anxiety and depression is essential for both caregivers and care recipients. Early detection and diagnosis can lead to effective treatment and improved quality of life. If you or your loved one are experiencing these symptoms, don't hesitate to seek professional help. Addressing these mental health challenges is a vital step toward a healthier and more balanced caregiving experience. In the next modules, we will explore practical strategies and treatments to manage anxiety and depression, helping you navigate your caregiving journey with resilience and strength.

Here's a funny quote about depression by comedian and writer Ruby Wax:

"If you are a depressive, you are a depressive not because you're lazy or not trying hard enough, but because your soul has the flu."

This quote highlights the serious nature of depression while using humor to convey the message that it is a condition that affects the mind just as the flu affects the body. Ruby Wax, known for her candid discussions about mental health, often uses humor to make the topic more approachable.

The Invisible Man
is Finally Seen

There once was an invisible carer, so kind,
But people would see him and not pay him mind.
They'd look right through him, like he wasn't there,
Unseen and unnoticed, he'd float through the air.

In silence he worked, with a heart full of care,
For those he looked after, he'd always be there.
But loneliness lingered, a shadow so wide,
No one could see the pain he held inside.

He'd smile and he'd nod, though his heart felt so cold,
Carrying burdens, both heavy and old.
Depression, a darkness, crept into his soul,
As he tended to others, it took quite a toll.

Invisible carer, his spirit would weep,
In the quiet of night, when the world was asleep.
He wished for a moment, for someone to see,
The struggles he faced, the silent plea.

His mind was a storm, with thoughts that would race,
But he'd show no trace, just a calm, steady face.
For those in his care, he gave all his might,
While inside he battled a constant night.

One day he met someone who seemed just like him,
A soul with a light that refused to grow dim.
She saw through his guise, to the sorrow he bore,
"You're not invisible," she said, "not anymore."

With a touch and a smile, she shared in his load,
Together they walked, down a new, brighter road.
The invisible carer, now seen and embraced,
Found comfort and peace, in a newfound place.

For sometimes it takes just one person to see,
The battles we fight, the silent plea.
Invisible no more, he found strength to share,
In the bonds of friendship, the power of care.

So, remember the carers who seem out of sight,
Their struggles are real, in the day and the night.
A kind word or gesture can brighten their way,
Turning the darkest of nights into day.

Remember:
There should never be such a thing
as an invisible carer!

CHAPTER 6

BUILDING RESILIENCE AND EMOTIONAL WELL-BEING

"Resilience is not just about bouncing back from adversity, but about thriving amidst the challenges. True well-being comes from nurturing our inner strength and embracing the journey with courage and grace."

6.1
Developing Resilience in Caregiving.

Introduction

Caregiving is a role filled with challenges, and developing resilience is key to navigating these difficulties while maintaining your own well-being. Resilience is the ability to bounce back from stress and adversity, a crucial skill for caregivers who often face physical, emotional, and mental demands. In this module, we will explore what resilience is, why it's essential in caregiving, and how you can cultivate this important trait by unlocking your inner abilities and superpowers.

Understanding Resilience

Resilience isn't about avoiding stress or never feeling overwhelmed. Instead, it's about how you respond to and recover from challenging situations. Resilient caregivers can adapt to the pressures of their role, maintain a sense of balance, and continue to provide effective care without sacrificing their own health. Resilience is like unlocking your superpowers, tapping into inner strengths and abilities you may not even realize you have.

Why Resilience Matters in Caregiving

Sustained Care: Resilience helps you sustain your caregiving efforts over the long term, reducing burnout and maintaining your ability to provide high-quality care.

Emotional Stability: It allows you to manage the emotional ups and downs of caregiving, preventing chronic stress and improving your mental health.

Problem-Solving: Resilient individuals are better equipped to handle unexpected challenges and find solutions to problems, enhancing their caregiving capabilities. Sometime's when solving problems, it is important to think outside the box.

Building Resilience: Key Strategies
Self-Awareness: Understanding your own emotions and triggers is the first step in building resilience. Regular self-reflection helps you recognize when you're becoming overwhelmed and allows you to take proactive steps to manage stress.

Positive Thinking: Maintaining a positive outlook can significantly impact your resilience. This doesn't mean ignoring difficulties but rather focusing on the positive aspects of caregiving, such as the difference you're making in your loved one's life. I mentioned earlier a personal story. Positve thinking is an important mindset to have. I found that my simply nodding to people when I speak really helps to contribute to a positive environment and it helps me think better. We will talk more about positive thinking later in this book.

Self-Care: Prioritizing self-care is crucial. This includes physical activities, hobbies, relaxation techniques, and ensuring you get enough rest. Remember, taking care of yourself is not selfish; it's necessary to be an effective caregiver.

Social Support: Building a network of supportive friends, family, and fellow caregivers can provide emotional backing and practical help. Don't hesitate to reach out for support when you need it.

Healthy Boundaries: Setting boundaries helps prevent caregiver burnout. Learn to say no to tasks that are beyond your capacity and seek help when needed. Establishing boundaries ensures you have time for your own needs and rest.

Flexibility and Adaptability: Being flexible allows you to adapt to changing circumstances and manage unpredictability better. Caregiving often involves unexpected situations, and a flexible mindset can help you handle these without undue stress.

POSITIVE THINKING

Maria's Journey to Resilience

Maria, a caregiver for her husband with multiple sclerosis, initially struggled with the overwhelming demands of caregiving. She often felt exhausted, both physically and emotionally. However, Maria decided to focus on building her resilience and unlocking her inner superpowers. She started by joining a caregiver support group, which provided her with a sense of community and understanding. This group became a vital source of emotional support and practical advice.

Maria also began practicing mindfulness meditation, spending a few minutes each day focusing on her breath and clearing her mind. This practice helped her manage stress and stay calm, even during the most challenging times. Additionally, Maria made a conscious effort to set boundaries, scheduling regular breaks and time for her hobbies, which rejuvenated her spirit and energy levels.

Through these efforts, Maria found that her ability to cope with the demands of caregiving improved significantly. She became more patient, less stressed, and better able to support her husband. Maria's journey to resilience demonstrates that with the right strategies and a focus on unlocking her superpowers, caregivers can thrive despite the challenges they face.

Questions for Self-Assessment

To understand your current level of resilience and identify areas for improvement, ask yourself the following questions:

- How do I typically react to stressful situations?
- Am I able to recognize when I'm becoming overwhelmed or stressed?
- Do I have a network of supportive friends or family members I can turn to for help?
- Do I regularly engage in activities that help me relax and recharge?
- How flexible am I in adapting to new or unexpected challenges?
- Do I practice positive thinking and focus on the positives in my caregiving role?
- What unique strengths do I bring to my caregiving role, and how can I develop these further?

Reflecting on these questions can help you identify strengths and areas where you may need to focus on building resilience and unlocking your caregiving superpowers.

Conclusion

Developing resilience is crucial for caregivers facing the relentless demands of their role. By understanding what resilience is and implementing strategies to enhance it, caregivers can better manage stress, maintain emotional stability, and continue providing compassionate care without sacrificing their own well-being. In the following modules, we will delve deeper into specific techniques and practices that can further support your journey towards resilience and emotional well-being. Remember, resilience is not about never feeling overwhelmed but about bouncing back and continuing to move forward, equipped with the tools and mindset to handle whatever comes your way. Embrace your inner abilities and superpowers to navigate the caregiving journey with strength and confidence.

6.2
Mindfulness and Sanity Checks

Introduction

In the whirlwind of caregiving, it's easy to lose sight of your own well-being. The constant demands can leave you feeling overwhelmed and disconnected from yourself. That's where mindfulness and regular sanity checks come in. These practices help you stay grounded, present, and balanced amidst the chaos. In this module, we will explore the concept of mindfulness and the importance of sanity checks, along with practical tips on how to incorporate them into your daily routine.

Understanding Mindfulness

Mindfulness is the practice of being fully present in the moment, aware of your thoughts, feelings, and surroundings without judgment. It's about observing your experiences as they are, without getting caught up in them. Mindfulness can be a powerful tool for caregivers, helping to reduce stress, increase emotional regulation, and improve overall well-being.

The Importance of Mindfulness in Caregiving

Stress Reduction: Mindfulness helps you manage stress by allowing you to step back from your worries and focus on the present moment. This can lower your overall stress levels and make caregiving more manageable.

Emotional Regulation: Being mindful helps you become more aware of your emotions and how they affect your behavior. This awareness can help you respond to challenging situations with greater calm and clarity.

Improved Focus: Mindfulness enhances your ability to concentrate, making it easier to stay focused on the task at hand and avoid becoming overwhelmed by the many responsibilities of caregiving.

Enhanced Well-being: Regular mindfulness practice has been shown to improve overall well-being, leading to a greater sense of peace, happiness, and fulfilment.

Incorporating Mindfulness into Your Routine

Start Small: Begin with just a few minutes of mindfulness practice each day. You can gradually increase the time as you become more comfortable with the practice.

Breathing Exercises: Simple breathing exercises can help you stay grounded. Try taking deep, slow breaths and focusing on the sensation of the air entering and leaving your body.

Mindful Observation: Take a moment to observe your surroundings. Notice the colours, sounds, and textures around you. This can help you feel more connected to the present moment.

Body Scan: A body scan involves paying attention to the sensations in different parts of your body, from your toes to your head. This can help you become more aware of physical tension and release it.

Mindful Activities: Engage in everyday activities mindfully. Whether it's eating, walking, or washing dishes, focus fully on the activity and notice the sensations and movements involved.

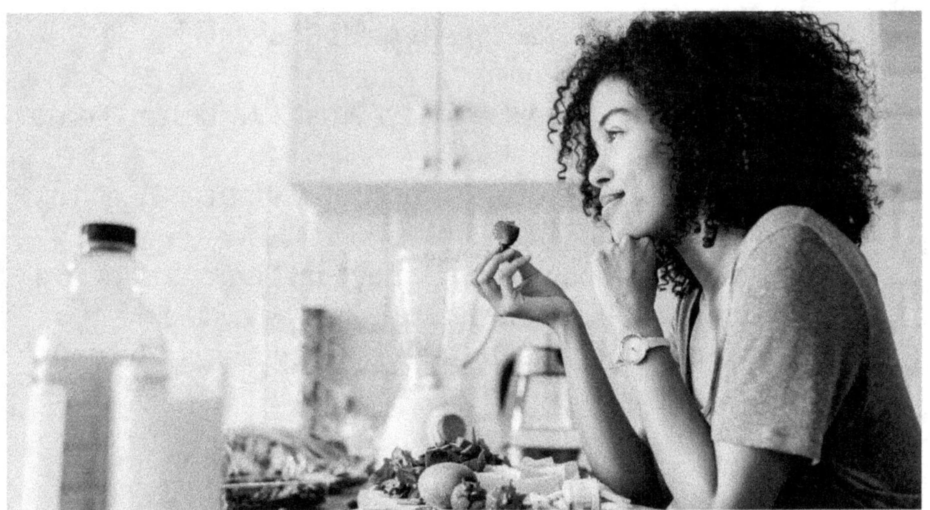

Sanity Checks: Reconnecting with Yourself

Sanity checks are regular self-assessments that help you stay in touch with your own needs and well-being. They are crucial for preventing burnout and ensuring that you remain healthy and balanced as a caregiver.

"All work and no play makes Jack a dull boy."

Why Sanity Checks are Important

Self-Awareness: Regularly checking in with yourself helps you stay aware of your mental and emotional state. This awareness allows you to address any issues before they become overwhelming.

Preventing Burnout: Sanity checks help you recognize when you're reaching your limits, so you can take steps to rest and recharge before you burn out.

Maintaining Balance: These checks ensure that you are taking time for yourself and maintaining a healthy balance between caregiving and self-care.

Questions for Your Sanity Checks

Here are some key questions to ask yourself.

- **Am I feeling overwhelmed or stressed?** If so, what is contributing to these feelings?
- **Have I taken time for myself today?** What activities can I do to relax and recharge?
- **Am I maintaining my social connections?** Who can I reach out to for support or companionship?
- **Are there hobbies or activities I enjoy that I haven't done in a while?** How can I make time for these in my schedule?
- **Am I getting enough rest and sleep?** What changes can I make to improve my rest?

Reconnecting with Your Passions

Do you remember the hobbies and activities that once brought you joy? Whether it's painting, gardening, reading, or playing an instrument, these activities are important for your mental health. Reconnecting with your passions can provide a much-needed escape from the demands of caregiving and help you recharge.

Schedule Time for Hobbies: Make a conscious effort to set aside time for activities you enjoy. Even a few minutes each day can make a difference.

Combine Hobbies with Caregiving: Find ways to incorporate your hobbies into your caregiving routine. For example, if you enjoy music, play your favourite songs while caring for your loved one.

Explore New Interests: Don't be afraid to try something new. Exploring new hobbies can bring excitement and novelty to your life, providing a mental and emotional boost.

Example: John's Sanity Checks and Mindfulness Practice

John, a caregiver for his mother with dementia, found himself constantly stressed and disconnected from his own needs. He decided to incorporate mindfulness and sanity checks into his routine. Each morning, John spent five minutes doing deep breathing exercises and a short body scan. He also scheduled weekly sanity checks, asking himself how he felt and what he needed to maintain his well-being.

John realized he missed his hobby of woodworking, which he had abandoned due to his caregiving responsibilities. He decided to set aside time each weekend to work on small projects. This not only gave him a sense of accomplishment but also provided a much-needed break from caregiving.

My Sanity Check: Papa Roy

Writing music has always been my sanctuary, my sanity check. When I was young, I played in bands, and the creative process of making music was deeply inspiring. It was an outlet for my emotions, a way to connect with others, and a source of immense joy. Several years later, I found my way back to writing music and invented my alter ego, "Papa Roy."

Creating music as Papa Roy is more than just a hobby; it's a crucial part of my mental well-being. Some people enjoy my music, while others may not, but for me, it's not about the approval. It's about the process, the creativity, and the sanity it brings me. It's my way of navigating life's ups and downs, a personal therapy that keeps me grounded.

If you're curious, you can find my music under 'Papa Roy' or 'Papa Roy Foundation' on Spotify and Apple Music. I also share my work on YouTube. Whether you're a fan or just curious, you're welcome to join me on this musical journey.

In creating and sharing my music, I maintain my mental health and stay connected to a part of myself that has always brought me peace, happiness and brought me a great deal of fun!

What's your sanity check?

Conclusion

Mindfulness and sanity checks are essential tools for caregivers to maintain their well-being and resilience. By staying present, reconnecting with your passions, and regularly assessing your needs, you can navigate the challenges of caregiving with greater ease and balance. Remember, taking care of yourself is not a luxury—it's a necessity. As you continue on your caregiving journey, let mindfulness and sanity checks guide you toward a healthier, more fulfilling experience.

Mindfulness is like crafting a recipe. You carefully consider all the ingredients to find ways to enhance the overall experience. Sometimes, everything blends perfectly, and it's about maintaining that balance and harmony.

6.3
The Power of Positive Thinking: Your Shield Against Kryptonite

In the demanding world of caregiving, positivity is not just a luxury—it's your superpower, your shield against the formidable challenges that come your way. By harnessing the power of positive thinking, you can fortify your emotional well-being, enhance your resilience, and navigate the twists and turns of the caregiving journey with strength and grace. In this module, we will explore the transformative effects of positive thinking, its role in maintaining emotional balance, and practical strategies for cultivating optimism in your daily life.

The Mighty Impact of Positive Thinking

Positive thinking isn't just about wearing rose-coloured glasses—it's about wielding a powerful shield against the adversities of caregiving. By adopting an optimistic mindset, you can turn obstacles into opportunities, setbacks into stepping stones, and challenges into catalysts for growth.

How Positive Thinking Protects You from Your Kryptonite

Reduced Stress:

Positive thinking acts as your Armor against stress, deflecting the blows of worry and anxiety. By focusing on the bright side of situations, you can dial down the tension and approach challenges with a calm, clear mind.

Enhanced Resilience:

Optimism is your secret weapon in the battle against adversity. With a positive outlook, you can bounce back from setbacks, adapt to changing circumstances, and emerge stronger than ever before.

Improved Emotional Well-being:
Positivity is your shield against the emotional onslaught of caregiving. By maintaining an optimistic attitude, you can safeguard your mental health, prevent burnout, and cultivate a sense of inner peace and contentment.

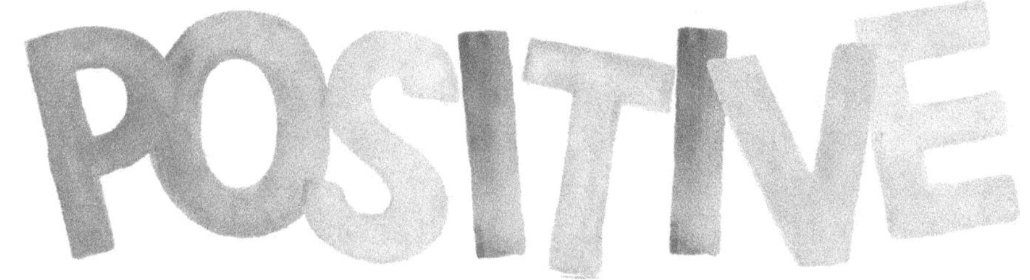

Practical Strategies for Embracing the Power of Positivity

Harness the Power of Gratitude: Armor yourself with gratitude by cultivating a daily practice of counting your blessings. Whether through journaling or silent reflection, take a moment each day to acknowledge the abundance in your life.

Challenge Negative Thoughts: Strengthen your shield against negativity by confronting and refuting negative thoughts as they arise. Replace self-doubt with self-affirmation, criticism with compassion, and despair with hope.

Visualize Victory: Envision success as your shield against defeat. Use the power of visualization to picture yourself overcoming challenges, achieving your goals, and emerging triumphant in the face of adversity.

Surround Yourself with Positivity: Forge alliances with fellow warriors of light—positive-minded individuals who uplift and inspire you. Seek out sources of positivity in your environment, from uplifting music to motivational literature, and bask in their radiant glow.

Focus on Solutions, Not Problems: Arm yourself with a problem-solving mindset by shifting your focus from obstacles to opportunities. Channel your energy into finding creative solutions to the challenges you encounter, and watch as your resilience grows.

IExamples of Positive Thinking as Your Shield

Finding Strength in Adversity: Like Superman confronting his greatest foe, a caregiver faces the challenges of caregiving with unwavering optimism. They see each obstacle as an opportunity for growth, each setback as a chance to rise stronger than before.

Maintaining Hope in the Face of Uncertainty: Just as Wonder Woman stands firm in the face of danger, a caregiver remains steadfast in their optimism, trusting in their ability to navigate the uncertainties of caregiving with grace and determination.

Embracing Joy in the Journey: Like Batman embracing the darkness with unwavering resolve, a caregiver embraces the joys and sorrows of caregiving with open arms. They understand that positivity is not the absence of challenges but the presence of resilience in the face of adversity.

Conclusion: Embrace the Power Within

In the epic saga of caregiving, positivity is your greatest ally, your stalwart companion in the face of adversity. By harnessing the power of positive thinking, you can shield yourself against the corrosive effects of stress, overwhelm, and despair. As you journey forward, remember that optimism is not just a mindset—it's a way of life, a beacon of hope in the darkest of times. Embrace the power within, and let positivity be your guiding light on the path to resilience and emotional well-being.

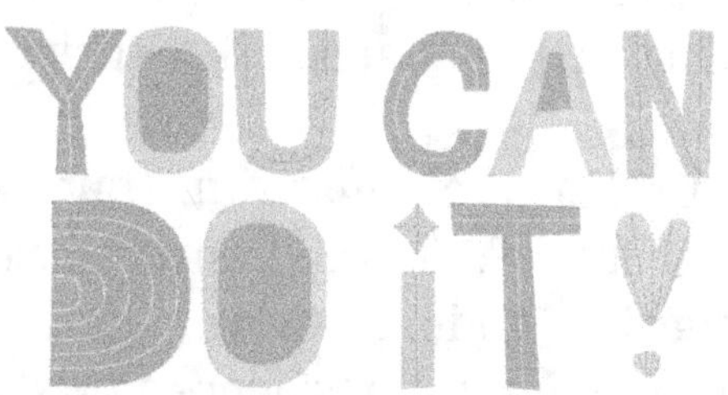

Captain Caring V The Evil D Mentia

Captain Caring, the hero of cheer,
Faced Evil D Mentia, who spread only fear.
With a cape of compassion and heart full of might,
Captain Caring vowed to set all things right.

D Mentia sneered with a villainous glare,
"Your kindness is weak, it doesn't compare!"
But Captain Caring, with a smile so wide,
Had tricks up his sleeve, and love on his side.

He tickled D Mentia with jokes and with jest,
And offered warm hugs to put him to rest.
"Your evil will falter, your gloom will collapse,
For nothing withstands my caring perhaps!"

D Mentia, bewildered, began to crack a grin,
His darkness receding, light seeping in.
"Fine, you win this round," D Mentia did say,
"But next time I'll bring more gloom to the fray!"

Captain Caring just laughed, "We'll see about that,
For kindness will triumph, and that is a fact!"
So off flew the hero, to spread more delight,
While D Mentia, now smiling, slunk into the night.

CHAPTER 7

PRACTICAL SELF-CARE STRATEGIES FOR CAREGIVERS

"Self-care is not a luxury; it's a necessity. Prioritize yourself, and watch how your strength and resilience inspire those around you."

7.1
Creating a Self-Care Routine

Caregiving is a demanding role that often leaves little time for personal well-being. However, prioritizing self-care is essential for maintaining your health, energy, and overall effectiveness as a caregiver. In this module, we will explore the importance of self-care, how to create a sustainable self-care routine, and practical strategies to ensure you remain balanced and resilient in your caregiving journey.

The Importance of Self-Care

Self-care is the practice of taking deliberate actions to maintain your physical, mental, and emotional health. For caregivers, self-care is not a luxury—it's a necessity. By taking care of yourself, you ensure that you have the strength and resilience needed to provide the best possible care for your loved one. Neglecting self-care can lead to burnout, compassion fatigue, and a decline in your own health, ultimately impacting your ability to care effectively.

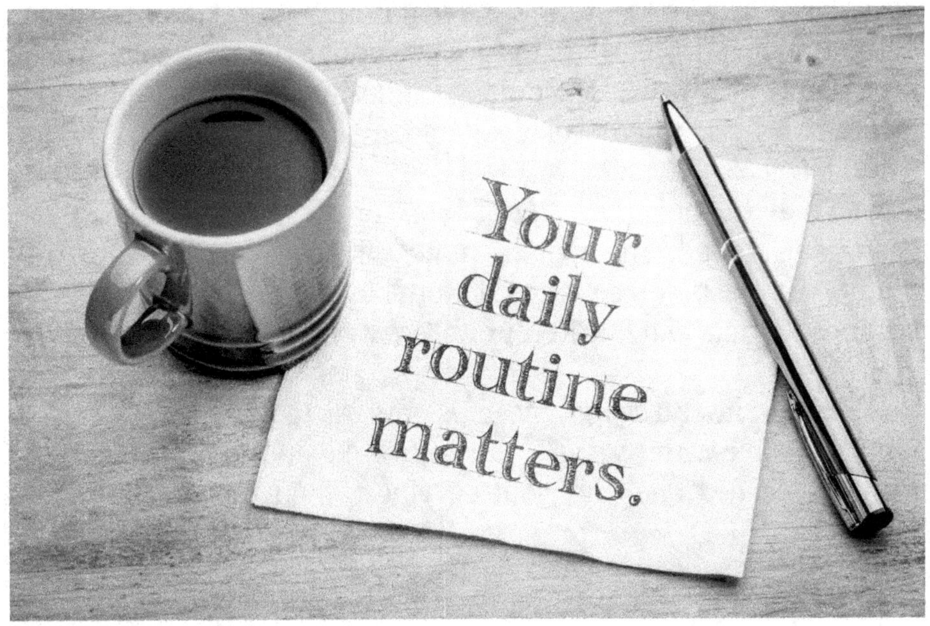

Steps to Creating a Self-Care Routine

Assess Your Needs: The first step in creating a self-care routine is to assess your current needs. Reflect on the areas of your life that require attention—physical health, mental well-being, emotional balance, and social connections. Identifying these areas will help you tailor a self-care routine that addresses your specific needs.

Set Realistic Goals: Establish realistic and achievable self-care goals. These goals should be specific, measurable, and tailored to fit into your daily life. For example, aim to incorporate 30 minutes of exercise into your routine three times a week or schedule a weekly coffee date with a friend.

Prioritize Self-Care Activities: Determine which self-care activities are most important to you and prioritize them. Consider activities that nourish your body, mind, and soul, such as exercise, meditation, hobbies, and social interactions. Make a list of these activities and incorporate them into your routine.

Create a Schedule: Develop a schedule that integrates self-care activities into your daily or weekly routine. Consistency is key to forming lasting habits, so try to allocate specific times for self-care. For instance, you might schedule a morning walk, an afternoon meditation session, or a weekly yoga class.

Start Small: If you're new to self-care, start with small, manageable changes. Gradually incorporate more self-care activities into your routine as you become more comfortable. Small steps can lead to significant improvements in your well-being over time.

Be Flexible: Life as a caregiver can be unpredictable, so it's essential to remain flexible with your self-care routine. Be prepared to adjust your plans as needed and give yourself grace when things don't go as planned.

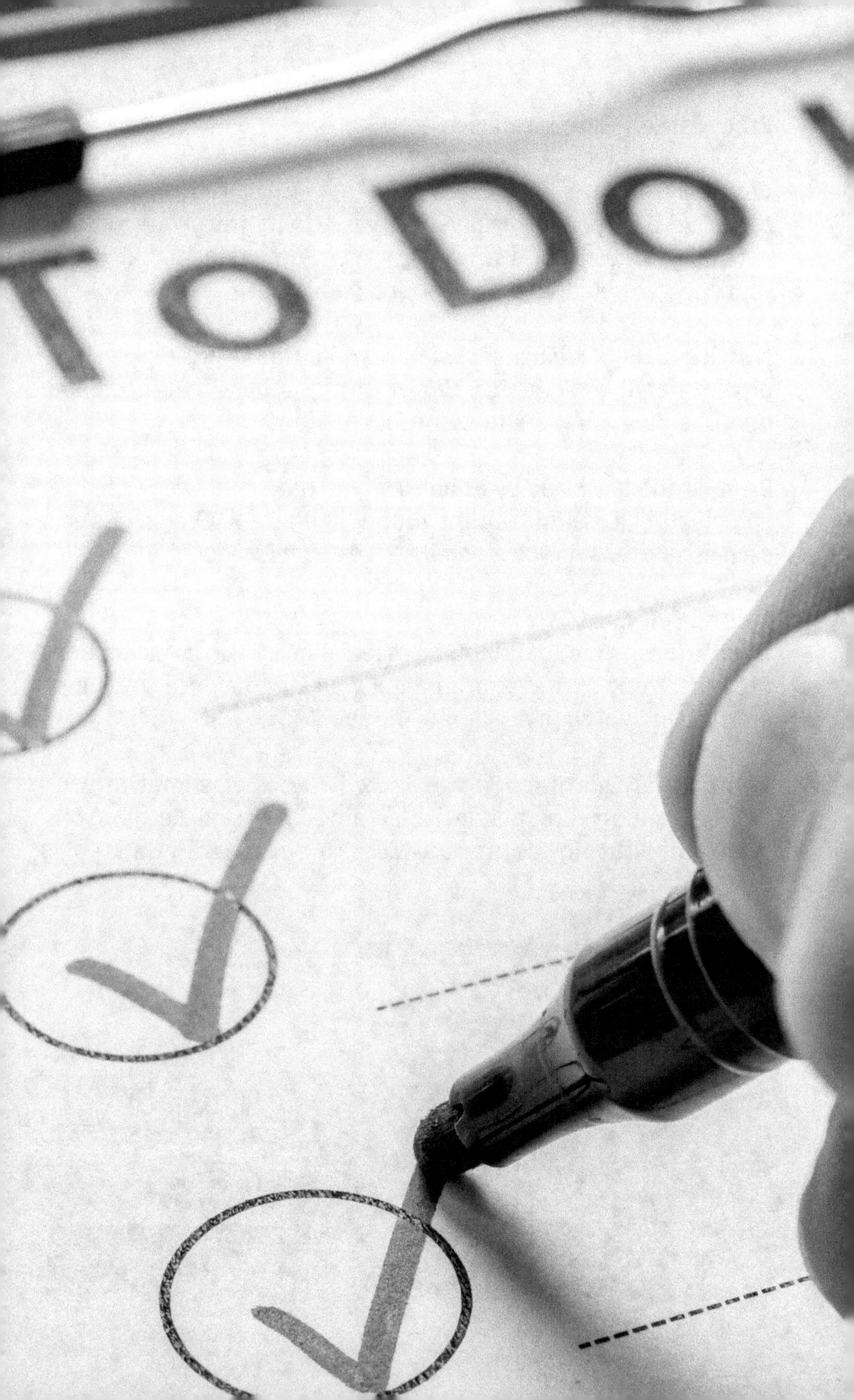

TO DO

Practical Self-Care Strategies

Physical Self-Care:
Exercise: Incorporate regular physical activity into your routine. Activities like walking, swimming, yoga, or even dancing can boost your energy levels and improve your mood.

Nutrition: Eat a balanced diet rich in fruits, vegetables, lean proteins, and whole grains. Proper nutrition fuels your body and mind, helping you stay strong and focused.

Sleep: Prioritize sleep by establishing a consistent sleep schedule and creating a restful bedtime routine. Aim for 7-9 hours of sleep each night to ensure you are well-rested and rejuvenated.

Mental Self-Care:
Mindfulness: Practice mindfulness techniques such as meditation, deep breathing exercises, or mindful walking to reduce stress and enhance mental clarity.

Continuous Learning: Engage in activities that stimulate your mind, such as reading, puzzles, or learning a new skill. Keeping your mind active can provide a mental escape from caregiving duties.

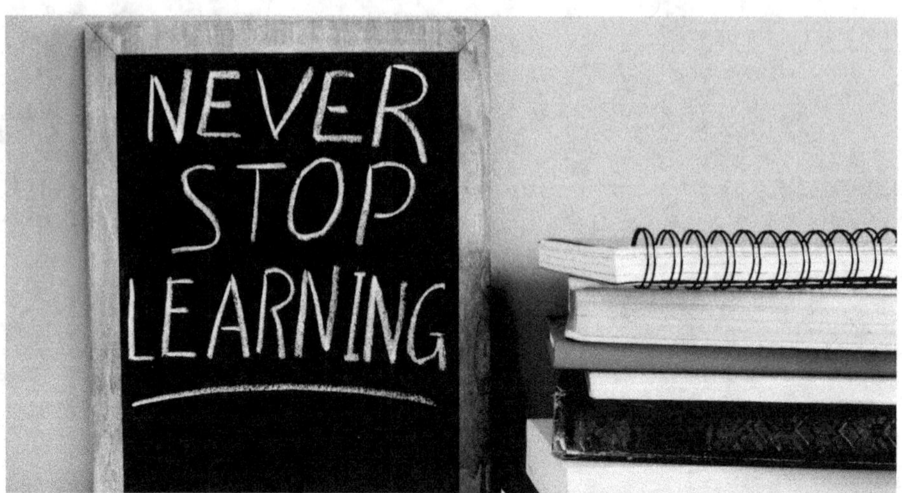

Emotional Self-Care:

Express Your Feelings: Find healthy outlets for your emotions, such as journaling, talking to a friend, or joining a support group. Expressing your feelings can help you process and manage stress.

Practice Self-Compassion: Be kind to yourself and acknowledge your efforts and achievements. Treat yourself with the same compassion and understanding that you offer to others.

Social Self-Care:

Connect with Others: Maintain social connections by spending time with friends and family. Engaging in social activities can provide emotional support and a sense of belonging.

Seek Support: Don't hesitate to seek help from others, whether it's through professional counselling, support groups, or respite care services. Building a support network can lighten your load and provide much-needed relief. There is support out there.

Many people are happy to subscribe monthly to satellite/ cable TV, or on a mobile phone contract. Why not subscribe in yourself and get the support you need. Yes, it may cost money but you are worth it!

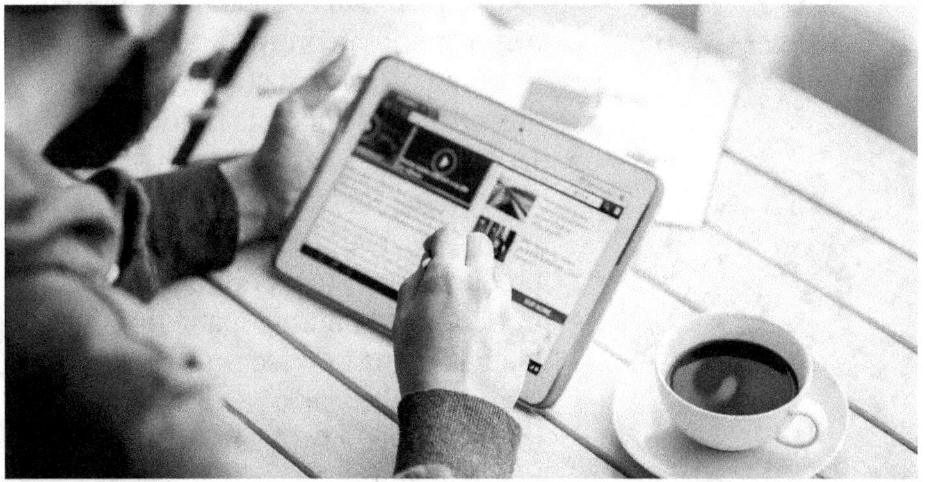

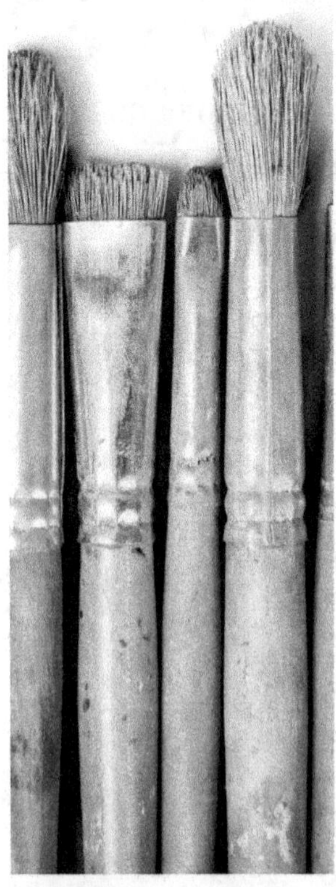

Self-Care Routine Ideas for Different Personalities

For the Creative Person:

- **Art and Craft Projects:** Set aside time each week for creative projects like painting, drawing, or crafting. These activities can provide a therapeutic escape and allow you to express yourself creatively.
- **Writing and Journaling:** Keep a journal or start writing short stories or poetry. This can be a wonderful outlet for your thoughts and emotions, helping you to process your experiences.
- **Music and Dance:** Engage in activities that involve music, whether it's playing an instrument, singing, or dancing. Music can be a powerful mood booster and stress reliever.

For the Practical-Minded Person:

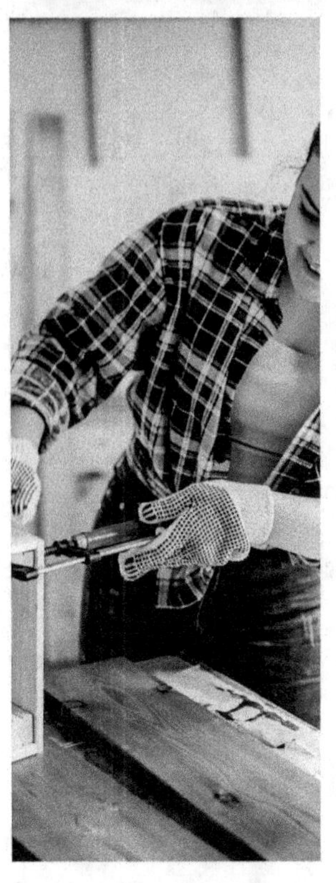

- **Organized Planning:** Create a detailed weekly plan that includes time for self-care activities. Using planners or digital tools can help you stay organized and ensure that you allocate time for yourself.
- **DIY Projects:** Take on small home improvement or DIY projects. These can provide a sense of accomplishment and a productive way to spend your downtime.
- **Cooking and Baking:** Spend time in the kitchen trying new recipes or baking treats. Cooking can be a relaxing and rewarding activity that nourishes both body and mind.

For the Hands-On Person:

- **Gardening:** Spend time in the garden planting, weeding, or simply enjoying the outdoors. Gardening can be both physically active and mentally soothing.
- **Exercise and Fitness:** Incorporate physical activities such as hiking, biking, or attending fitness classes. Staying active is crucial for your physical and mental health.
- **Volunteer Work:** Engage in volunteer activities that allow you to give back to the community. This can provide a sense of purpose and fulfillment beyond your caregiving duties.

Combination of all person:

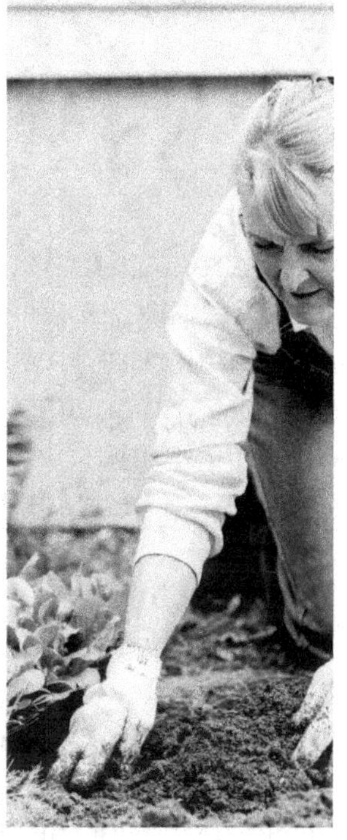

- **Love you pet!:** Having a pet can help. It is something you can do on your own, or socially and animals provide a great deal of comfort.
- **Group activities:** Join a group, running club or local society. This can be done either online, or face to face.

Conclusion

Creating a self-care routine is a vital component of effective caregiving. By prioritizing your well-being, you equip yourself with the strength, resilience, and emotional balance needed to provide compassionate and sustainable care for your loved one. Remember, self-care is not selfish —it's an essential investment in your health and the quality of care you provide.

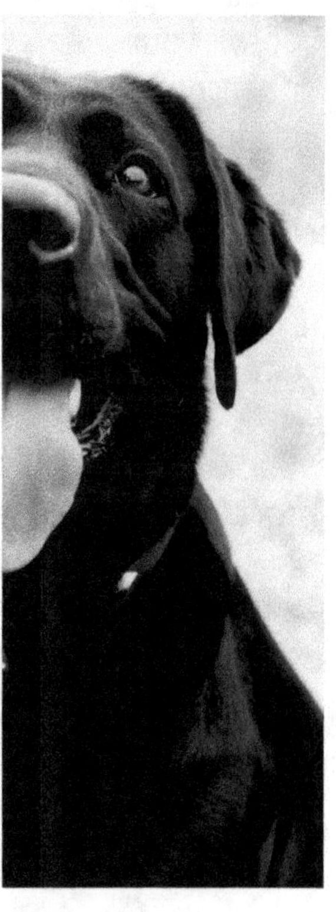

7.2
Nutrition, Exercise, and Sleep

As a caregiver, maintaining your physical health is crucial to providing the best care for your loved one. Nutrition, exercise, and sleep are the three pillars of physical well-being, and they play an essential role in keeping you energised, focused, and resilient. This module will explore the importance of a balanced diet, regular exercise, and quality sleep, along with practical tips to incorporate these elements into your daily routine. Remember, by prioritizing your health, you are better equipped to care for others, and reading this book is a testament to your commitment to self-care.

The Importance of a Balanced Diet
A balanced diet provides the essential nutrients your body needs to function optimally. As part of your routine, you can create dishes to include these. I for one have found cooking a great Sanity Check! It boosts your energy levels, supports your immune system, and enhances your overall well-being. Here are some key points to consider:

Nutrient-Rich Foods:
Fruits and Vegetables: These are packed with vitamins, minerals, and antioxidants that help protect your body from illness. Aim to fill half your plate with a variety of colourful fruits and vegetables.

Whole Grains: Foods like brown rice, quinoa, and whole-wheat bread provide sustained energy and are rich in fibre, which aids digestion.

Lean Proteins: Incorporate lean meats, fish, eggs, beans, and nuts into your diet to help repair tissues and maintain muscle mass.
Healthy Fats: Include sources of healthy fats, such as avocados, nuts, seeds, and olive oil, which support brain health and hormone production.

Healthy Fats: Include sources of healthy fats, such as avocados, nuts, seeds, and olive oil, which support brain health and hormone production.

Hydration: Drinking enough water is vital for maintaining energy levels and overall health. Aim for at least 8 glasses of water a day and adjust according to your activity level and climate.

Regular Meals and Snacks: Eating regular, balanced meals and healthy snacks helps maintain stable blood sugar levels, preventing energy slumps and mood swings.

The Importance of Exercise

Regular physical activity is essential for maintaining your physical and mental health. Exercise releases endorphins, which improve mood and reduce stress. Here are some simple ways to incorporate exercise into your daily routine:

Walking: Walking is a low-impact, accessible form of exercise that can be easily incorporated into your day. Aim for at least 30 minutes of walking most days of the week. You can break this into shorter, more manageable sessions if needed.

Example: *Take a brisk walk around your neighbourhood, park further from store entrances, or use the stairs instead of the elevator.*

Stretching and Flexibility Exercises: Stretching helps maintain flexibility and reduce muscle tension. Incorporate a few minutes of stretching exercises into your morning or bedtime routine. I have found that this helps to relieve the tension from your back muscles, and it has helped me to look after my lower back.

Example: *Try simple stretches like touching your toes, side stretches, or yoga poses like the cat-cow stretch or child's pose.*

Strength Training: Building muscle strength helps support your joints and maintain mobility. You don't need a gym membership—bodyweight exercises like squats, lunges, and push-ups can be done at home.

Example: Incorporate strength training exercises into your routine two to three times a week, using household items like water bottles as weights if needed.

Activity Breaks: If your caregiving duties keep you busy, take short activity breaks throughout the day. Even a few minutes of movement can make a difference.

Example: Set a timer to remind yourself to stand up, stretch, or take a quick walk every hour.

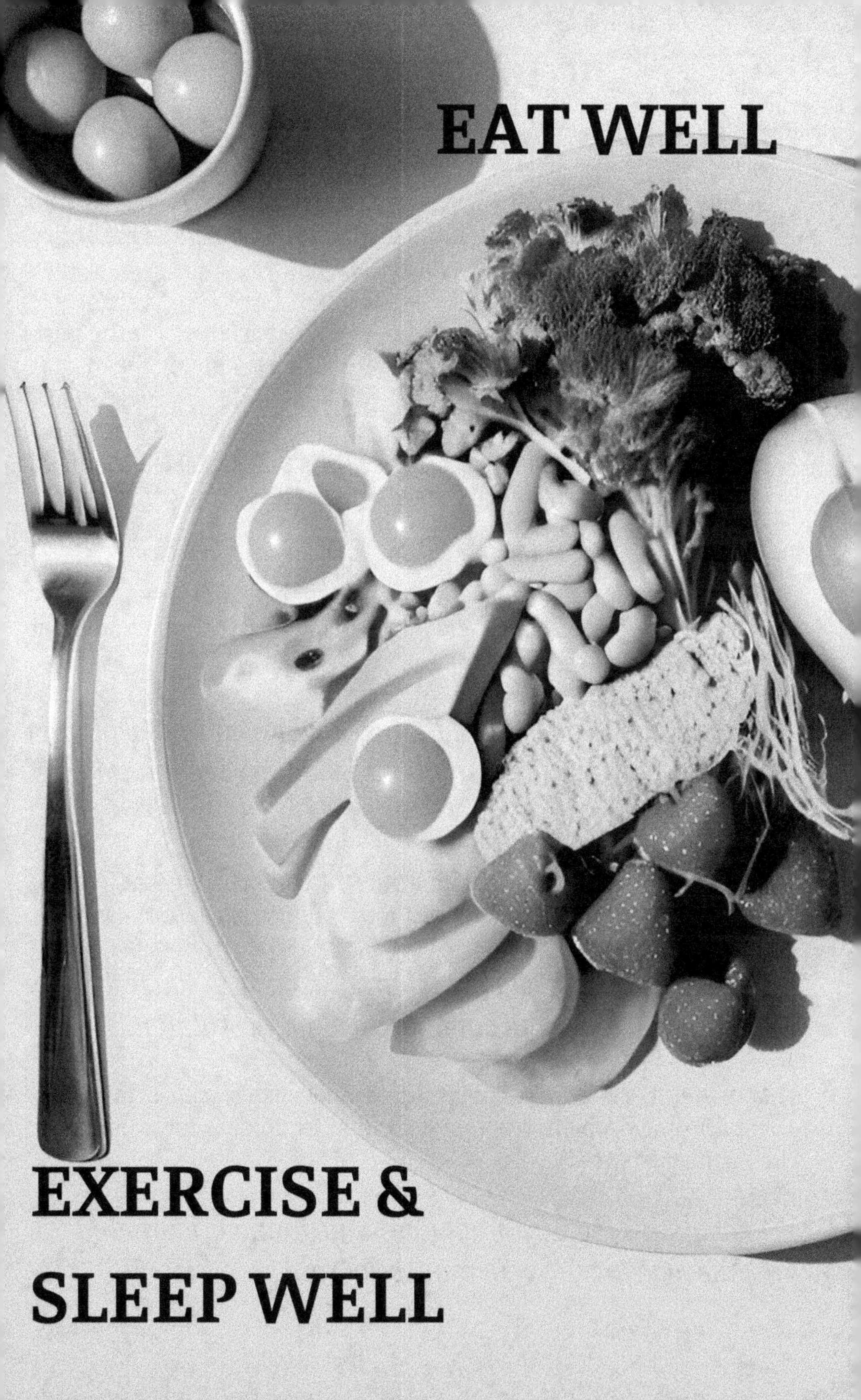

EAT WELL
EXERCISE &
SLEEP WELL

The Importance of Sleep

Quality sleep is vital for physical and mental health. It allows your body to repair itself and your mind to process emotions and memories. Here are some tips to improve your sleep quality:

Establish a Sleep Routine: Going to bed and waking up at the same time each day helps regulate your internal clock. Aim for 7-9 hours of sleep each night.

Example: Create a relaxing bedtime routine that signals to your body it's time to wind down, such as reading a book, taking a warm bath, or practicing deep breathing exercises.

Create a Restful Environment: Ensure your bedroom is conducive to sleep. Keep it cool, dark, and quiet, and invest in a comfortable mattress and pillows.

Example: *Use blackout curtains, a white noise machine, or earplugs to eliminate disruptions, and keep electronic devices out of the bedroom.*

Limit Stimulants: Avoid caffeine, nicotine, and heavy meals close to bedtime, as they can interfere with your ability to fall and stay asleep.

Example: *opt for a light, calming snack if you're hungry before bed, like a small banana or a handful of almonds.*

Manage Stress and Anxiety: Stress and anxiety can significantly impact your sleep. Incorporate relaxation techniques into your day to help manage stress levels.

Example: *Practice mindfulness meditation, journaling, or gentle yoga to calm your mind before bed.*

Conclusion

Maintaining a balanced diet, regular exercise, and quality sleep are foundational to your well-being as a caregiver. By incorporating these elements into your daily routine, you not only enhance your health and resilience but also set a positive example for those you care for. Remember, self-care is a continuous journey, and making small, consistent changes can lead to significant improvements in your overall health and caregiving experience. Embrace these strategies, prioritize your well-being, and continue to invest in yourself as you navigate the rewarding and challenging role of caregiving.

7.3
Finding Time for Yourself

Tic Tok- Time is ticking!
One of the most common challenges caregivers face is finding time for themselves amidst their demanding responsibilities. The phrase "I haven't got time" often becomes a mantra, but it's crucial to shift this mindset. Self-care is not a luxury; it is essential for your health and well-being. This module will emphasize the importance of making time for yourself and provide practical strategies to help you do just that.

Why Making Time for Yourself is Crucial
As a caregiver, your days are filled with tasks and responsibilities, leaving little room for personal time. However, neglecting your own needs can lead to burnout, reduced effectiveness in caregiving, and even health issues. By making time for yourself, you can recharge, reduce stress, and maintain a positive outlook, which benefits both you and the person you care for.

Common Barriers to Self-Time
Guilt: Many caregivers feel guilty taking time for themselves, believing that all their time should be devoted to their loved ones.

Overwhelm: The sheer volume of caregiving tasks can make it seem impossible to carve out personal time.

Lack of Support: Without adequate support, caregivers may struggle to find time away from their duties.

You and MYSELF: Sometimes you can be the biggest barrier to Self-Time. Take the time out!

Shifting the Mindset: Make Time, Don't Find Time
The key to self-care is to make time, not just find time. This proactive approach requires a shift in mindset and the understanding that self-care is a priority, not an option. Here are some strategies to help you make time for yourself:

Schedule It In: Treat self-care like any other appointment. Block out time on your calendar specifically for activities that rejuvenate you.

Example: *Schedule a 30-minute walk in the morning or a relaxing bath in the evening.*

Delegate Tasks: Don't hesitate to ask for help. Delegate caregiving tasks to family members, friends, or professional caregivers to free up some time for yourself.

Example: *Ask a neighbour to stay with your loved one for an hour while you take a break.*

Use Respite Care: Take advantage of respite care services that provide temporary relief for caregivers. This can give you a few hours or even days to focus on yourself.

Example: *Enrol your loved one in a day program once a week to give yourself a break.*

Incorporate Self-Care into Daily Routines: Look for opportunities to integrate self-care into your existing routines.

Example: *Practice deep breathing exercises while waiting for appointments or listen to your favourite music while cooking dinner.*

Scenario 1: *Maria, a full-time caregiver for her mother, felt constantly overwhelmed and guilty about taking any time for herself. By scheduling a weekly yoga class and arranging for a neighbour to sit with her mother during that time, Maria was able to recharge and found that her overall mood and energy levels improved.*

Scenario 2: John, who cares for his wife with dementia, struggled to find any personal time. He began by setting small, manageable goals such as taking a 15-minute coffee break each afternoon. Gradually, he incorporated longer breaks by using respite care services, which greatly reduced his stress.

Conclusion

Making time for yourself is not a selfish act—it is a critical component of effective caregiving. By prioritizing self-care, you enhance your ability to provide compassionate and sustainable care for your loved one. Implement these strategies to create personal time in your daily routine and witness the positive impact on both your well-being and your caregiving experience. Remember, by investing in yourself, you are also investing in the quality of care you provide.

"There once was a carer named Leigh,
Who cared for folks tirelessly.
But she learned self-care's key,
Took a break, felt so free,
Now she smiles as she's
made time for a wee!"

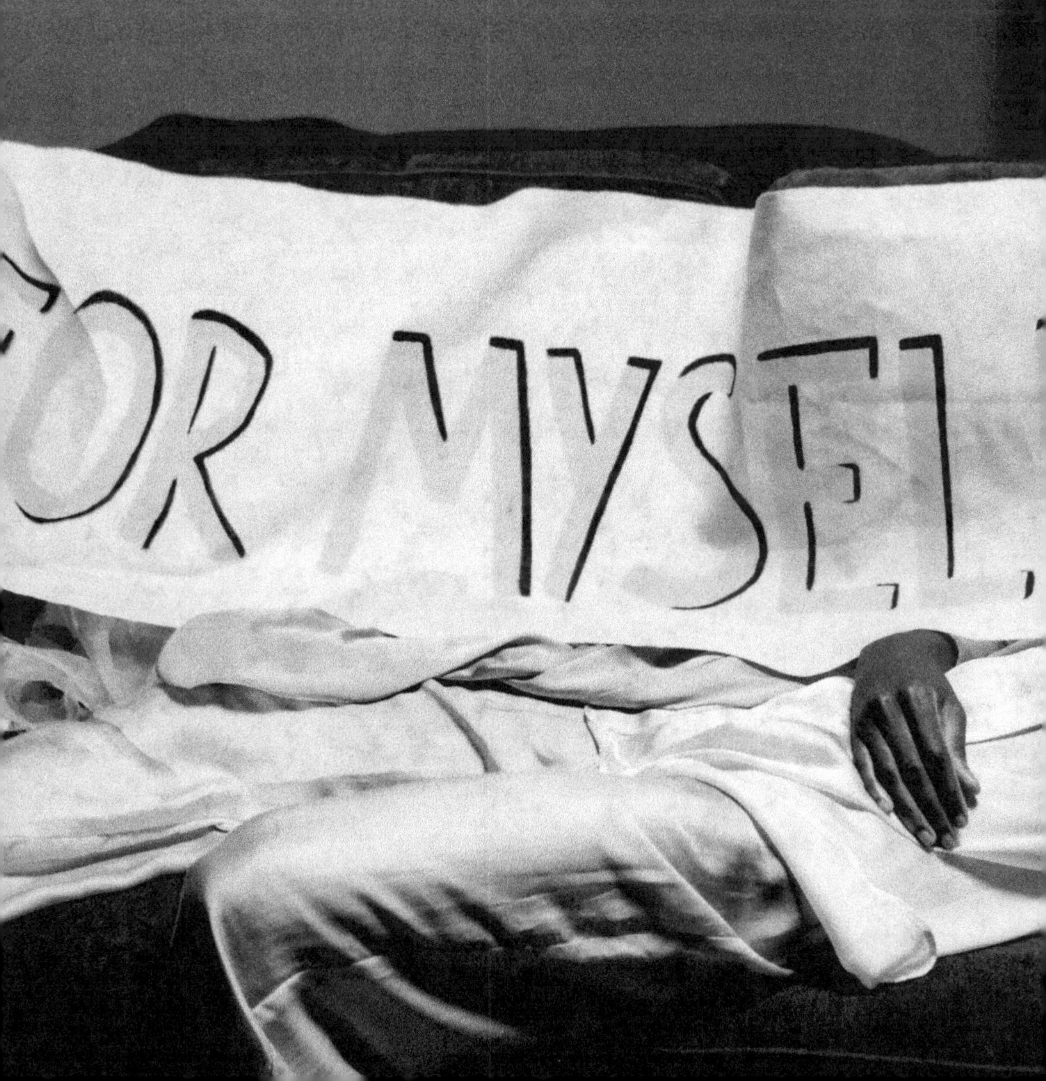

Batman and Catwoman: Wellness Warriors

In Gotham's dark, where villains roam,
Batman and Cat woman found their home.
But amidst the chaos, they needed a break,
Time together, for their sanity's sake.

So off they went, to a hidden retreat,
where they could relax and kick up their feet.
No capes, no gadgets, just laughter and fun,
In the warm glow of the setting sun.

Cat woman donned a dress of red,
While Batman traded black for blue instead.
They danced and they sang, feeling so free,
No worries, no crimes, just them and the sea.

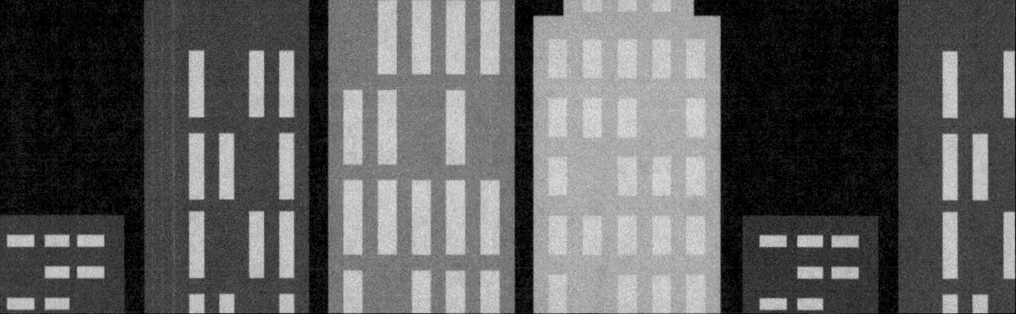

But they also knew, to stay at their best,
they needed more than just leisure and rest.
So, they ate nutritious meals, filled with delight,
Fuelling their bodies for the day and the night.

Exercise was important, they both agreed,
so they jogged on the beach,
planting each seed Of health and vitality, in their
bodies so strong,
as they ran, they sang their superhero song.

And when the stars twinkled, signalling night,
they nestled in bed, snuggling tight.
For sleep was essential, for body and mind, R
charging their spirits, in dreams so kind.

So, here's to Batman and his feline friend,
Balancing heroics with self-care, to no end.
For in nurturing themselves, they find the key,
to continue protecting Gotham, happy and free.

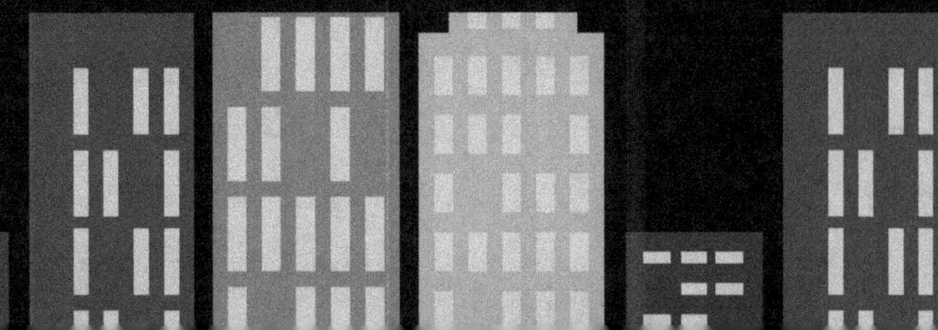

CHAPTER 8

EFFECTIVE COMMUNICATION AND RELATIONSHIPS

8.1
Communicating with Loved Ones

Effective communication is the foundation of successful caregiving. Whether you are caring for a loved one with complex needs, learning difficulties, dementia or autism, learning to communicate effectively can significantly enhance your caregiving experience. This module will explore the importance of communication, the challenges posed by various conditions, and strategies to improve your interactions with those you care for and with other family members and friends.

Why Effective Communication Matters

Communication is crucial in caregiving for several reasons:

Building Trust and Understanding: Clear and compassionate communication helps build trust between you and your loved one. It ensures that their needs, preferences, and concerns are understood and addressed.

Reducing Misunderstandings and Frustrations: Effective communication minimizes misunderstandings and reduces frustrations, leading to a more harmonious caregiving environment.

Ensuring Safety and Well-being: Good communication is essential for conveying important information about health, medication, and daily activities, which ensures the safety and well-being of your loved one.

Strengthening Relationships: Open and honest communication strengthens relationships with other family members and friends, fostering a supportive network for caregiving.

"Communication is like acting and you need to adapt yourself to the audience!"

Challenges in Communication

Communicating with loved ones who have certain conditions can be challenging. Understanding these challenges is the first step toward improving communication.

Complex Needs: Individuals with complex medical conditions may have difficulty expressing their needs clearly. They may rely on non-verbal cues, which can be easily misinterpreted.

Learning Difficulties: People with learning difficulties may struggle with understanding and processing information, requiring more patience and simpler language.

Autism: Those with autism may have unique communication styles, including difficulty with social cues, eye contact, and expressive language. They may also prefer routines and specific ways of interaction.

Dementia: As their condition worsens, you need to adapt yourself in order to communicate. Often they may regress into themselves and their mind transfers back in time. They may be referring to their mother or father, long since departed. You may need to enter their world when you communicate to act in their best interests.

Strategies for Effective Communication

Active Listening: Truly listen to your loved one without interrupting. Show empathy and understanding by acknowledging their feelings and concerns.

Example: *If your loved one with autism is upset, listen to their concerns without immediately offering solutions. This shows respect for their feelings.*

Use Simple and Clear Language: Use straightforward language and short sentences. Avoid jargon or complex terms that may confuse your loved one.

Example: *Instead of saying, "We need to monitor your dietary intake to manage your diabetes," say, "We need to watch what you eat to keep your blood sugar in check."*

Non-Verbal Communication: Pay attention to body language, facial expressions, and gestures. These can provide valuable clues about how your loved one is feeling.

Example: *If a non-verbal loved one with complex needs points to a specific area, investigate what they might need or want in that context.*

Patience and Repetition: Be patient and willing to repeat information as needed. Some individuals may need extra time to process what you are saying.

Example: *When explaining a new routine to someone with learning difficulties, repeat the instructions calmly and use visual aids if possible.*

Strategies for Effective Communication
Active Listening: Truly listen to your loved one without interrupting. Show empathy and understanding by acknowledging their feelings and concerns.

Example: *If your loved one with autism is upset, listen to their concerns without immediately offering solutions. This shows respect for their feelings.*

Use Simple and Clear Language: Use straightforward language and short sentences. Avoid jargon or complex terms that may confuse your loved one.

Example: *Instead of saying, "We need to monitor your dietary intake to manage your diabetes," say, "We need to watch what you eat to keep your blood sugar in check."*

Non-Verbal Communication: Pay attention to body language, facial expressions, and gestures. These can provide valuable clues about how your loved one is feeling.

Example: *If a non-verbal loved one with complex needs points to a specific area, investigate what they might need or want in that context.*

Patience and Repetition: Be patient and willing to repeat information as needed. Some individuals may need extra time to process what you are saying.

Example: *When explaining a new routine to someone with learning difficulties, repeat the instructions calmly and use visual aids if possible.*

Use Visual Aids and Tools: Visual aids, such as pictures, charts, and written instructions, can be helpful, especially for those with learning difficulties or autism. Example: Create a daily schedule with pictures for a loved one with autism to help them understand and anticipate their daily activities.

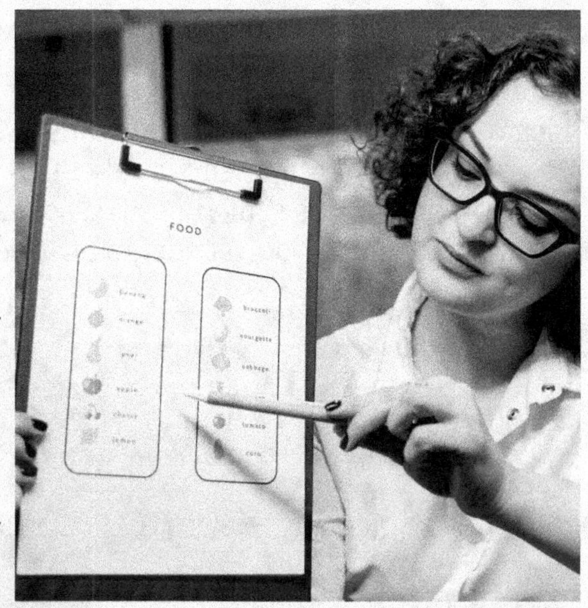

Example: *Create a daily schedule with pictures for a loved one with autism to help them understand and anticipate their daily activities.*

Create a Calm Environment: Minimize distractions and create a calm environment to improve focus and understanding during conversations.

Example: *Turn off the TV and other noise when having a discussion with your loved one.*

Empathy and Validation: Show empathy and validate your loved one's feelings and experiences. This fosters a sense of being heard and understood.

Example: *If your loved one with complex needs expresses frustration, acknowledge their feelings by saying, "I understand this is frustrating for you."*

Communicating with Family Members and Friends

Apologises in advance for swearing, but I am now going to use the word family. Effective communication extends beyond your loved one to include family members and friends. Maintaining open lines of communication with them is essential for a cohesive caregiving support system. This sometimes is a source of conflict and irritation, but it is important you get this right. This is a swear word to some people.

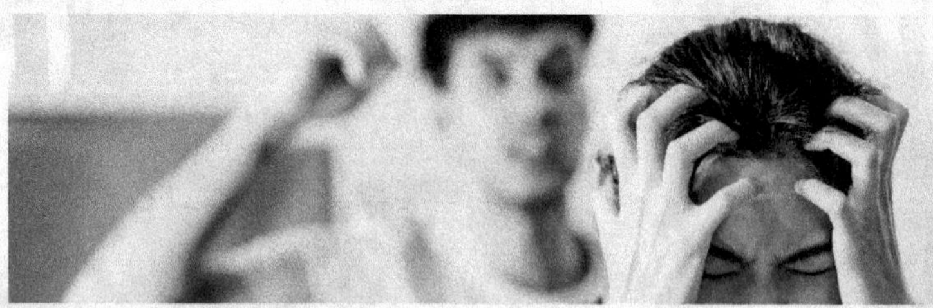

Regular Updates: Keep family members and friends informed about the loved one's condition, progress, and any changes in care plans.

Example: *Send regular emails or set up a family group chat to share updates and important information.*

Express Needs Clearly: Clearly communicate your needs and limits as a caregiver to family and friends. Ask for specific help when needed.

Example: *If you need a break, say, "I need someone to stay with [Loved One] for a few hours on Saturday so I can have some personal time."*

Involve Them in Care: Involve other family members and friends in caregiving tasks, decisions, and activities. This can reduce your burden and foster a sense of shared responsibility.

Example: *Assign specific tasks to willing family members, such as grocery shopping, meal preparation, or taking your loved one to appointment.*

Conflict Resolution: Address conflicts and disagreements openly and constructively. Focus on finding solutions rather than assigning blame.

Example: *If a disagreement arises about the best care approach, hold a family meeting to discuss everyone's perspectives and reach a consensus.*

Emotional Support: Lean on your support network for emotional support. Sharing your experiences and feelings can help reduce stress and prevent burnout.

Example: *Schedule regular check-ins with a close friend or family member to talk about your caregiving journey and express any concerns or frustrations.*

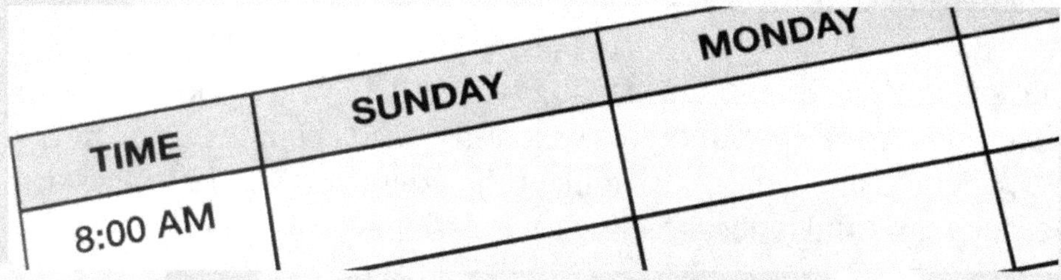

Conclusion

Effective communication is a cornerstone of successful caregiving. By learning to communicate clearly and empathetically with your loved one and maintaining open lines of communication with family and friends, you can build a supportive and harmonious caregiving environment. Remember, communication is not just about talking; it's about listening, understanding, and connecting. Embrace these strategies to enhance your caregiving experience and strengthen your relationships.

8.2
Building a Support Network

We have talked about support network earlier, so hear is a few extra tips. Building a robust support system is not just about having a safety net—it's about creating a lifeline that sustains you through the challenges and celebrates your triumphs. This module will delve into the importance of cultivating a support network and provide inspiration to motivate you on this empowering endeavour.

Why Building a Support Network Matters
Strength in Numbers: A support network provides strength and resilience, offering multiple shoulders to lean on during difficult times. When you have a network of people rooting for you, no challenge seems insurmountable.

Emotional Wellness: Connecting with others who understand your journey can be incredibly validating and comforting. Sharing experiences and feelings with like-minded individuals fosters a sense of belonging and reduces feelings of isolation.

Practical Assistance: Your support network can offer practical assistance, whether it's helping with caregiving tasks, providing respite care, or offering guidance and resources. Knowing you have a team behind you can ease the burden of caregiving responsibilities.

Empowerment and Motivation: Surrounding yourself with supportive individuals empowers you to advocate for your needs and those of your loved one. Their encouragement and motivation fuel your determination to overcome obstacles and pursue your caregiving journey with resilience and grace.

The Power of Your Support Network

In the realm of caregiving, as in the world of superheroes and iconic teams, the strength of unity knows no bounds. Just as the Fantastic Four, the A-Team, Charlie's Angels, and the crew of the Starship Enterprise accomplished remarkable feats through collaboration, so too can caregivers achieve greatness together. When individuals join forces, their collective efforts become a force to be reckoned with. Together, they can overcome challenges, conquer obstacles, and accomplish extraordinary things. While we may draw inspiration from fictional characters in this book, remember that you have the power to make your own team come to life. With unity, resilience, and unwavering support, there is no limit to what you can accomplish together.

8.3
Navigating Difficult Conversations

Difficult conversations are an inevitable part of the caregiving journey, but they are also opportunities for growth, understanding, and resolution. Whether you're speaking with the person you're supporting, healthcare professionals, or care providers, navigating these conversations with empathy and clarity is essential. This module will explore strategies for handling difficult conversations and provide examples of scenarios where these conversations may arise.

Who You May Have Difficult Conversations With

The Person You're Supporting:
Discussing sensitive topics such as changes in care needs, medical decisions, or end-of-life preferences can be challenging but necessary.

Healthcare Professionals or Experts:
Conversations with healthcare professionals may involve seeking clarification on medical conditions, discussing treatment options, or advocating for your loved one's needs.

Care Providers:

Communicating with care providers about expectations, concerns, or issues related to the quality of care requires diplomacy and assertiveness.

Family:
Sorry, I swore again! These, however, can be very difficult. They may not see all the hard work and support you have been giving. It is important you show them this.

Strategies for Navigating Difficult Conversations

Prepare in Advance: Take time to prepare for the conversation by clarifying your goals, gathering relevant information, and anticipating potential challenges or objections.

Choose the Right Time and Place: Select a time and place that is conducive to open communication and free from distractions. Ensure privacy and minimize interruptions.

Listen Actively: Practice active listening by giving the speaker your full attention, acknowledging their perspective, and refraining from interrupting or rushing to respond.

Express Yourself Clearly and Empathetically: Use clear and concise language to express your thoughts and feelings. Speak with empathy and sensitivity, considering the other person's emotions.

Seek Common Ground: Look for areas of agreement or shared interests to build rapport and foster cooperation. Focus on finding solutions that benefit all parties involved.

Stay Calm and Respectful: Remain calm and composed, even if the conversation becomes heated or emotional. Avoid blaming or criticizing others and maintain a respectful tone.

Acknowledge Emotions: Validate the other person's emotions and acknowledge their concerns or fears. Demonstrating empathy can help de-escalate tense situations and facilitate understanding.

Focus on Solutions: Keep the conversation focused on finding constructive solutions or compromises rather than dwelling on past grievances or assigning blame.

Follow Up: After the conversation, follow up with any agreements or action items discussed. Reiterate your commitment to ongoing communication and collaboration.

Navigating Family Conflicts

Once again, I would like to apologise for swearing again! Here's more about family! Family conflicts are often at the heart of caregiving challenges. Loved ones may struggle to accept changes in their family member's health or abilities, leading to disagreements and strained relationships. When addressing family conflicts:

Recognize Different Perspectives: Understand that family members may have differing views and experiences that shape their perceptions of the situation.

Communicate with Empathy: Approach conversations with empathy and understanding, acknowledging the emotions and concerns of all parties involved.

Clarify Misunderstandings: Address any misunderstandings or misconceptions about the caregiving situation, providing clear and information to promote understanding.

Focus on Shared Goals: Emphasize the importance of working together towards shared goals, such as the well-being and comfort of the person receiving care.

Seek Mediation if Needed: If conflicts persist, consider seeking the assistance of a neutral third party, such as a counsellor or mediator, to facilitate productive discussions and resolution.

Remember their way of looking: With conditions such as dementia, the family may remember them as they were, not for whom they have become and changed into. Dealing with things on a day to day basis can be challenging and they may not realise what has happened I always recommend keeping a journal of everything you do..

Conclusion

Difficult conversations are an inevitable aspect of caregiving, but with patience, empathy, and effective communication strategies, they can lead to greater understanding and collaboration. By employing these strategies and addressing family conflicts with compassion and respect, you can navigate challenging situations and foster harmony within your caregiving team.

To some people, families can be a swear word. To some they can be a fantastic support network. It's important that you all see the big picture to support THE OTHER ONE.

Remember, your ultimate goal is to provide the best possible care for your loved one while maintaining supportive relationships with those around you.

Dear Carer

Dear Carer, I want you to know, In my world, words may not flow. Autistic, they say, with a unique mind, Communication's a challenge, hard to find.

But within this struggle, there's a light, A hope that shines, burning bright. Though words may fail, and silence reign, There's a deeper language, without refrain.

Through art, through touch, through melody, I find my voice, I find my glee. With your patience and understanding, we'll rise above, Navigating this world with courage and love.

So please, dear carer, heed my plea, in my silence, there's more to see. With acceptance and kindness, we'll thrive, our bond unbreakable, as we strive.

CHAPTER 9

PROFESSIONAL HELP & RESOURCES

"Being a mental health professional is like being a human GPS: we help you navigate your mind's back roads, avoid the emotional potholes, and never judge when you take a detour for snacks!"

9.1
When to Seek Professional Help

Caregiving is a demanding role that often requires a wide range of skills and emotional resilience. While many caregivers manage the challenges they face with grace and determination, there are times when seeking professional help becomes necessary. Recognizing when to reach out for additional support can make a significant difference in both the caregiver's well-being and the quality of care provided. This module will explore the signs that indicate it might be time to seek professional help, the types of professionals who can assist, and how to approach this important decision.

Recognizing When to Seek Professional Help
Overwhelming Stress and Burnout: If you find yourself feeling constantly overwhelmed, exhausted, and unable to cope with the demands of caregiving, it may be time to seek help. Chronic stress and burnout can lead to serious health issues, both physically and mentally.

Persistent Feelings of Anxiety or Depression: Experiencing ongoing feelings of anxiety, depression, or hopelessness that interfere with your daily life and caregiving duties is a clear signal that professional help is needed. Mental health professionals can provide the support and treatment necessary to manage these conditions.

Decline in Physical Health: Neglecting your own health due to caregiving responsibilities can result in a decline in physical well-being. If you are experiencing frequent illnesses, unexplained aches and pains, or significant weight changes, consulting a healthcare professional is crucial.

Relationship Strain: Caregiving can put a strain on relationships with family and friends. If conflicts and communication issues are becoming more frequent and intense, seeking guidance from a family therapist or counsellor can help improve these dynamics.

Inability to Provide Adequate Care: When the needs of your loved one surpass your ability to provide appropriate care, it's time to consider professional help. This could involve hiring in-home care providers, seeking respite care, or exploring long-term care options.

Behavioural Changes in the Care Recipient: Significant changes in the behaviour or condition of the person you are caring for, such as increased aggression, confusion, or a sudden decline in health, may require professional assessment and intervention.

Safety Concerns: If you are concerned about the safety of your loved one or yourself, whether due to physical limitations, cognitive decline, or environmental hazards, professional help can provide solutions and support to ensure a safe caregiving environment.

Types of Professional Help

Healthcare Professionals: Doctors, nurses, and specialists can provide medical care, conduct assessments, and offer treatments for both caregivers and care recipients.

Mental Health Professionals: Therapists, counsellors, and psychologists can offer support for managing stress, anxiety, depression, and other mental health issues. They can also provide strategies for coping and improving emotional well-being.

Social Workers: Social workers can assist with navigating the healthcare system, accessing community resources, and providing emotional support and counselling.

Care Managers: Professional care managers can help develop and coordinate care plans, connect you with appropriate services, and provide ongoing support and advocacy.

In-Home Care Providers: Home health aides, personal care aides, and nurses can provide direct care and assistance with daily activities, allowing caregivers to take necessary breaks.

Respite Care Services: Respite care offers temporary relief for primary caregivers by providing short-term care for their loved ones, either in-home or at a dedicated facility.

Care Coaches and Trainers: These professionals are a valuable source of support for caregivers, providing advice, coaching, and support tailored to individual needs. While you have to pay for this type of service (just like a lawyer or private doctor), it is worth using their services. After all, people are willing to pay for satellite TV services; this is an investment in yourself and your well-being. They have often worked in care and trained in care settings, so they are able to relate to your situations better.

Approaching the Decision

Assess Your Needs: Take an honest assessment of your current situation, including your physical and emotional health, the needs of the care recipient, and the resources available to you.

Research Options: Explore the various types of professional help available and consider which options best meet your needs and those of your loved one. Look into the qualifications, experience, and reviews of potential providers.

Consult with Others: Discuss your thoughts and concerns with trusted family members, friends, or other caregivers who may have faced similar situations. Their insights and support can be invaluable.

Start Small: If you are hesitant about seeking professional help, start with small steps, such as attending a support group, scheduling a consultation with a therapist, or arranging for short-term respite care.

Communicate Openly: When you decide to seek professional help, communicate openly with the care recipient and other family members. Explain the reasons for your decision and how it will benefit everyone involved.

Conclusion

Recognizing when to seek professional help is a crucial aspect of effective caregiving. By paying attention to the signs of stress, burnout, and declining health, and by exploring the various types of professional support available, you can ensure that both you and your loved one receive the care and assistance needed. Remember, seeking help is not a sign of weakness, but a proactive step towards providing the best possible care and maintaining your own well-being. As you continue reading this book, you will find more strategies and resources to support you on your caregiving journey.

9.2
Types of Mental Health Professionals

Navigating the mental health landscape can be daunting, especially for caregivers who are already juggling numerous responsibilities. Understanding the different types of mental health professionals available can help you find the right support for both yourself and the person you are caring for. This module will provide an overview of various mental health professionals, including therapists, counsellors, psychologists, psychiatrists, social workers, and care coaches and trainers. Each of these professionals offers unique expertise and services that can significantly enhance your caregiving experience.

Therapists

Therapists, also known as psychotherapists or counsellors, are trained to help individuals deal with a wide range of emotional and psychological issues. They use various therapeutic techniques to address mental health conditions, improve coping skills, and support emotional well-being.

Licensed Professional Counsellors (LPCs): These professionals have advanced degrees in counselling and are licensed to diagnose and treat mental health conditions. They often focus on specific areas such as grief, trauma, or family therapy.

Marriage and Family Therapists (MFTs): MFTs specialize in relationships and family dynamics. They can help caregivers manage the emotional strain that caregiving places on family relationships.

Overall Therapists can be expensive, however they offer vital support and many care givers have benefitted from them.. It's worth investing in yourself we you need to.

Psychologists

Psychologists hold doctoral degrees in psychology (Ph.D. or Psy.D.) and are experts in diagnosing and treating mental health conditions. They use a variety of therapeutic approaches, such as cognitive-behavioural therapy (CBT), to help individuals manage their mental health.

Clinical Psychologists: They focus on assessing and treating mental health disorders through psychotherapy. They can provide valuable support for caregivers dealing with anxiety, depression, and other mental health challenges.

Neuropsychologists: These specialists focus on how brain injuries or illnesses impact behaviour and cognitive functions. They can be particularly helpful for caregivers of individuals with dementia, brain injuries, or other neurological conditions.

Psychiatrists

Psychiatrists are medical doctors (MDs) who specialize in diagnosing, treating, and preventing mental health disorders. They can prescribe medication and provide therapy. Their medical training allows them to understand the complex interplay between physical and mental health.

General Psychiatrists: They treat a broad range of mental health conditions and can provide medication management alongside psychotherapy.

Geriatric Psychiatrists: Specializing in the mental health of older adults, they can offer insights and treatments for age-related mental health issues, which is particularly relevant for caregivers of elderly individuals.

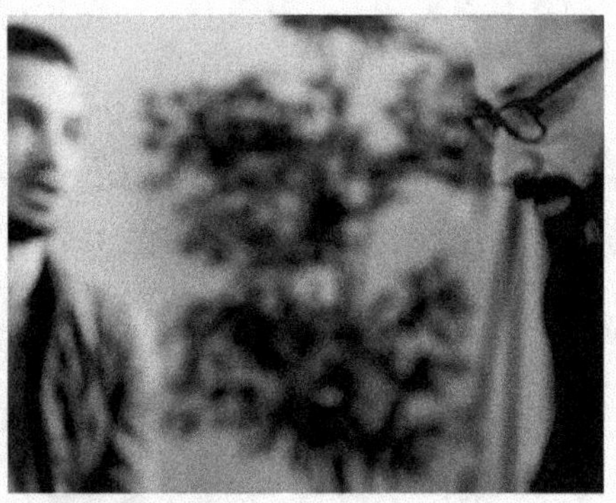

Social Workers

Social workers with a focus on mental health, often referred to as clinical social workers, provide counselling and support to individuals dealing with a variety of challenges.

Licensed Clinical Social Workers (LCSWs): They are trained to provide psychotherapy and counselling services. They can help caregivers access community resources, develop care plans, and provide emotional support.

Medical Social Workers: They work in healthcare settings and help patients and families navigate the complexities of the healthcare system. They can be invaluable in coordinating care and connecting caregivers with necessary services.

Care Coaches and Trainers

While not strictly mental health professionals, care coaches and trainers offer relevant support from a healthcare perspective. They provide practical advice, coaching, and training tailored to the unique challenges faced by caregivers.

Care Coaches: These professionals work with caregivers to develop personalized care plans, improve caregiving skills, and manage stress. They offer a supportive, non-judgmental space to discuss challenges and find solutions.

Trainers: Trainers often conduct workshops and courses on various aspects of caregiving, including mental health, communication skills, and practical care techniques. They equip caregivers with the knowledge and tools needed to provide high-quality care.

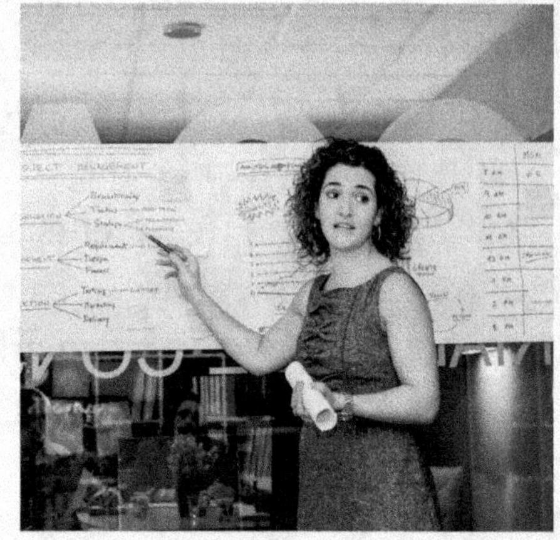

Conclusion

Understanding the roles of different mental health professionals can help you make informed decisions about the support you need. Whether it's therapy, medication management, or practical advice from care coaches, each type of professional brings valuable expertise to the table. As you continue your caregiving journey, don't hesitate to seek out the appropriate support to enhance both your well-being and that of the person you care for. Remember, utilizing these resources is a proactive step towards effective caregiving and maintaining your own mental health.

9.3
Accessing Community Resources

Community resources can provide invaluable support to caregivers, offering everything from practical assistance to emotional support. Knowing where to find and how to access these resources can significantly ease the burden of caregiving. This module will guide you through the various community resources available in the United Kingdom, the United States, Canada, and Australia. It will also provide strategies for identifying and utilizing these resources effectively. For detailed lists of resources specific to each country, refer to the appendix at the end of this eBook.

United Kingdom
In the UK, a variety of community resources are available to support caregivers. These include government programs, non-profit organizations, and local support groups.

1. **National Health Service (NHS):** The NHS offers a range of services for caregivers, including respite care, counselling, and support groups. The NHS Carers Direct helpline provides information and advice on all aspects of caregiving.
2. **Carers UK:** A leading charity that provides support, information, and advocacy for caregivers. They offer a helpline, online forums, and local support groups.
3. **Age UK:** This organization offers resources for caregivers of older adults, including advice on navigating the healthcare system, financial support, and respite care options.
4. **Local Authorities:** Many local councils provide support services for caregivers, including assessments, care plans, and access to local resources. Contact your local council's social services department for more information.

United States

The US offers a wide array of resources through federal programs, state initiatives, and non-profit organizations.

1. **Family Caregiver Alliance (FCA):** This organization provides information, support, and resources for caregivers, including online tools, fact sheets, and support groups.
2. **AARP Caregiving Resource Centre:** Offers a wealth of information and tools for caregivers, including guides, webinars, and a community forum.
3. **National Alliance for Caregiving (NAC):** Provides research, policy analysis, and advocacy for caregiver support. They also offer resources and connections to local support services.
4. **Local Area Agencies on Aging (AAA):** These agencies offer services for older adults and their caregivers, including respite care, meal delivery, and support groups. Find your local AAA through the Eldercare Locator.

Canada

In Canada, caregivers can access a variety of resources through federal and provincial programs, as well as non-profit organizations.

1. **Canadian Caregiver Coalition:** A national body that provides information, advocacy, and resources for caregivers. Their website offers a comprehensive directory of services and supports.
2. **Alzheimer Society of Canada:** Offers resources for caregivers of individuals with dementia, including support groups, educational materials, and a helpline.
3. **Provincial Caregiver Organizations:** Many provinces have their own caregiver support organizations, such as Caregivers Nova Scotia and the Ontario Caregiver Organization, which provide localized support and resources.
4. **Health Canada:** Offers information on federal programs and benefits available to caregivers, including financial assistance and respite care.

Australia

Australia provides numerous resources for caregivers through government programs, non-profit organizations, and community groups.

1. **Carers Australia:** The national peak body representing carers. They offer a range of services, including counselling, advocacy, and support groups.
2. **My Aged Care:** A government portal providing information on aged care services, including respite care, in-home care, and residential care options.
3. **Dementia Australia:** Offers support for caregivers of individuals with dementia, including a helpline, support groups, and educational resources.
4. **Local Carer Support Services:** Many local communities have carer support organizations that offer practical assistance, support groups, and respite care. Contact your local council for more information.

Strategies for Accessing Community Resources

1. **Research and Reach Out:** Start by researching the available resources in your area. Use online directories, helplines, and community centres to gather information. Don't hesitate to reach out directly to organizations for guidance.
2. **Connect with Other Caregivers:** Join support groups or online forums to connect with other caregivers. They can offer first-hand advice and recommendations on useful resources.
3. **Utilize Healthcare Providers:** Talk to your healthcare provider about available resources. They can often refer you to local services and support networks.
4. **Advocate for Yourself and Your Loved One:** Don't be afraid to ask for help and advocate for the services you need. Be persistent in seeking out the best possible support.
5. **Stay Informed:** Keep up to date with new programs and services by subscribing to newsletters, following relevant organizations on social media, and attending community events.

Conclusion

Accessing community resources is a crucial aspect of effective caregiving. These resources provide essential support, alleviate the burden on caregivers, and enhance the quality of care for your loved one. By utilizing the services available in your country, you can ensure that you and your loved one receive the necessary assistance and support. For more detailed lists of resources in the UK, US, Canada, and Australia, refer to the appendix at the end of this eBook.

Henry Viii
& His Care Cutbacks

Henry the Eighth, with his regal air, Was not a man known for tender care. Six wives he took, in search of delight, But his caregiving skills were far from right.

Catherine of Aragon, loyal and true, Faced a king who didn't have a clue. When no son came, his patience did drop, "Divorce her!" he cried. Care cutbacks, chop!

Anne Boleyn, with her wit and charm, Soon found herself in grave harm. False charges flew, the axe did drop, Her head rolled away. Chop, chop, chop!

Jane Seymour, sweet and fair, Died giving birth, but did Henry care? He moved on swiftly, didn't even stop, Her memory fading. Care cutbacks, chop!

Anne of Cleves, a political pawn, Saw her marriage over before the dawn. "Too plain," said Henry, with a heartless flop, Annulled and discarded. Care cutbacks, chop!

Catherine Howard, young and wild, Soon found herself in Henry's files. Accused of treason, she couldn't swap, Her fate was sealed. Chop, chop, chop!

Catherine Parr, the final queen, Outlived the king, but it was seen, Henry's care was cut back, leaving her to mop, Cleaning up his mess. Care cutbacks, chop!

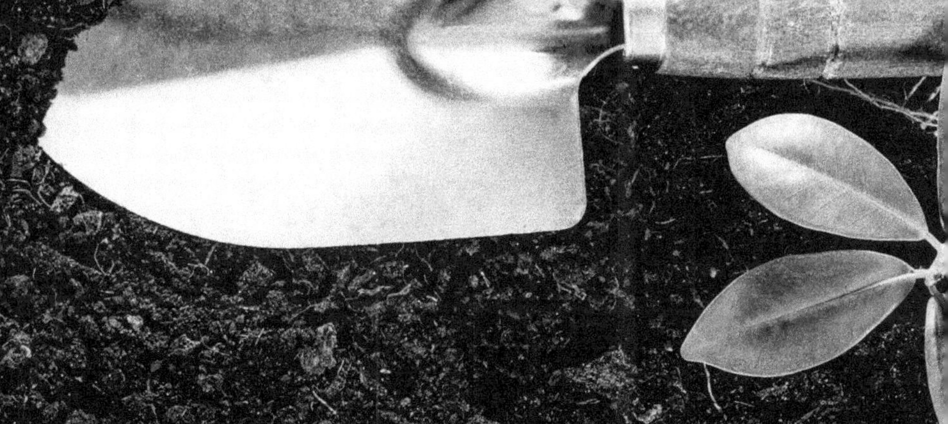

CHAPTER 10

ADDRESSING MENTAL HEALTH NEEDS IN THE OTHER ONE

"Taking care of someone's mental health is like being a gardener for their mind – sometimes you need to water, sometimes you need to prune, and sometimes you just need to let them bask in the sunshine of your company!"

10.1
THE OTHER ONE and Understanding Challenging Behaviours!

When caring for a loved one, especially someone with mental health needs, it's easy to focus on the visible, often challenging behaviours without recognizing the underlying causes. This can lead to frustration and exacerbate the situation for both the caregiver and the care recipient. In this module, we'll explore how to address the mental health needs of those you support, identify underlying issues that may be driving challenging behaviours, and develop strategies for creating a supportive and understanding environment.

Understanding Challenging Behaviours

Challenging behaviours, often referred to as "red zones," can include aggression, withdrawal, irritability, and other actions that disrupt daily life. While it's natural to react to these behaviours, it's crucial to look beyond them to understand their root causes.

Aggression and Agitation: Causes: Aggression and agitation can stem from pain, discomfort, confusion, or fear. For example, a person with dementia might become aggressive if they are unable to communicate their needs or if they feel threatened by an unfamiliar environment.

Impact: These behaviours can create a stressful environment, leading to increased tension between the caregiver and the care recipient.

Withdrawal and Depression

Causes: Withdrawal and depression may result from feelings of isolation, loss of independence, or the side effects of medication. Chronic illnesses and cognitive decline can also contribute to these feelings.

Impact: Withdrawal can make caregiving more challenging, as the caregiver may struggle to engage the patient in necessary activities.

Anxiety and Restlessness

Causes: Anxiety and restlessness are often linked to fear of the unknown, changes in routine, or sensory overload. Individuals with autism, for instance, may become anxious in new or crowded environments.

Impact: Anxiety can lead to behaviours like pacing, repetitive actions, or verbal outbursts, which can be distressing for both the caregiver and the care recipient.

Identifying Underlying Causes

To effectively address mental health needs, it's essential to identify the underlying causes of challenging behaviours. This requires a combination of observation, communication, and collaboration with healthcare professionals.

Observation

Patterns and Triggers: Observe the care recipient's behaviour to identify patterns and triggers. Note the times of day, specific activities, or environmental factors that precede challenging behaviours.

Physical Health: Monitor for signs of physical discomfort, such as grimacing, restlessness, or changes in eating and sleeping patterns. Pain or discomfort can often manifest as challenging behaviours.

Communication

Open Dialogue: Maintain open and honest communication with the care recipient, if possible. Encourage them to express their feelings and concerns. For non-verbal individuals, pay attention to non-verbal cues like body language and facial expressions.

Validation: Validate their feelings and experiences. Acknowledge their emotions without judgment, which can help reduce anxiety and build trust.

Collaboration with Healthcare Professionals
Multidisciplinary Approach: Work with a team of healthcare professionals, including doctors, psychologists, and social workers, to develop a comprehensive understanding of the care recipient's mental health needs.

Regular Assessments: Schedule regular mental health assessments to monitor changes and adjust care plans accordingly.

Addressing Specific Mental Health Needs
Different mental health conditions require tailored approaches to care. Understanding these conditions can help caregivers provide more effective support.

Dementia
Approach: Use clear, simple communication and provide step-by-step instructions for tasks. Create a calm environment and avoid sudden changes that can cause confusion.

Support: Engage in activities that stimulate cognitive function, such as puzzles, music therapy, and reminiscence therapy. Even though they may have dementia, they still are people and they need you!

Autism
Approach: Establish clear routines and provide visual aids to support communication. Be mindful of sensory sensitivities and create a sensory-friendly environment. Autism is a complex subject. The A and the U, I have always said stands for always unique.

Support: Encourage social interaction and communication through structured activities and positive reinforcement. Positive support has worked well for me in this area and it really works! Any support should always be person centred and taylored to the person's needs and wishes.

Acquired Brain Injury (ABI)

Approach: Provide consistent, repetitive training to help relearn skills. Use assistive devices to support independence.

Support: Engage in cognitive rehabilitation activities and offer emotional support to cope with changes in abilities.

Learning Difficulties

Approach: Use clear, concise language and break tasks into manageable steps. Provide hands-on guidance and support.

Support: Foster a supportive learning environment with tailored educational resources and activities.

Cerebral Palsy

Approach: Provide consistent, repetitive training to help relearn skills. Use assistive devices to support independence.

Support: Engage in cognitive rehabilitation activities and offer emotional support to cope with changes in abilities.

Conclusion

Addressing the mental health needs of care recipients is crucial for their well-being and the effectiveness of caregiving. By understanding the underlying causes of challenging behaviours and tailoring care to specific mental health conditions, caregivers can provide compassionate and effective support. Remember, the goal is to look beyond the "red zones" and address the root causes of behaviour, ultimately improving the quality of life for both the caregiver and the care recipient. For more resources and detailed strategies, refer to the appendix at the end of this eBook.

Example: Addressing Aggression in Dementia

Consider the case of Mary, a caregiver for her husband John, who has dementia. John often becomes aggressive in the late afternoon, a phenomenon known as "sundowning." Mary initially reacted with frustration, which escalated John's aggression. After observing John's behaviour patterns and consulting with a healthcare professional, Mary discovered that John's aggression was linked to fatigue and sensory overload.

These changes helped reduce John's aggression and improved their relationship, making caregiving more manageable for Mary.

Remember: People can be
challenging but you can always
be amazing!

10.2 Creating a Supportive Environment

Creating a supportive environment is essential for the well-being of both care recipients and caregivers. A well-designed environment can significantly reduce stress, enhance mood, and improve the overall quality of life. This module explores various strategies to create a supportive environment that benefits both the care recipient and the caregiver.

Understanding the Care Recipient's Needs

The first step in creating a supportive environment is understanding the specific needs and preferences of the care recipient. This involves recognizing their physical, emotional, and cognitive requirements.

Personal Preferences: Involve the care recipient in decisions about their environment whenever possible. This can include choosing colours, furniture, and personal items that make them feel comfortable and at home.

Sensory Needs: Consider sensory sensitivities, particularly for individuals with conditions like autism or dementia. This might involve reducing noise levels, using soft lighting, or incorporating calming scents.

Physical Environment Adjustments

Adjusting the physical environment can greatly impact the comfort and safety of the care recipient.

Safety Modifications: Ensure that the living space is safe and accessible. This might include installing grab bars in the bathroom, using non-slip mats, and arranging furniture to prevent falls.

Comfortable Living Space: Create a cosy and welcoming space by using comfortable furniture, soft blankets, and pillows. Personalize the space with photos, artwork, and other items that are meaningful to the care recipient.

Creating Routine and Structure

Routine and structure provide a sense of stability and predictability, which can be particularly beneficial for individuals with cognitive impairments.

Daily Schedules: Establish a daily routine that includes regular mealtimes, activities, and rest periods. Consistency helps reduce anxiety and confusion.

Visual Aids: Use visual aids like calendars, clocks, and daily schedules to help the care recipient understand and anticipate daily activities.

Emotional Support

Creating an emotionally supportive environment is crucial for the mental well-being of the care recipient.

Positive Communication: Use positive and encouraging language. Acknowledge the care recipient's feelings and provide reassurance when they are anxious or upset.

Social Interaction: Encourage social interaction with family members, friends, and other caregivers. Social connections can reduce feelings of isolation and loneliness.

Engaging the Senses

Engaging the senses can have a calming and therapeutic effect on care recipients.

Music Therapy: Use music that the care recipient enjoys to create a soothing atmosphere. Music can evoke positive memories and improve mood.

Aromatherapy: Introduce calming scents like lavender or chamomile through diffusers or scented candles.

Tactile Stimulation: Provide items that offer tactile stimulation, such as soft blankets, textured pillows, or fidget toys.

Technology and Assistive Devices

Technology and assistive devices can enhance the care recipient's independence and comfort.

Smart Home Technology: Use smart home devices to control lighting, temperature, and entertainment systems, making it easier for the care recipient to manage their environment.

Assistive Devices: Utilize assistive devices like hearing aids, mobility aids, and communication devices to support the care recipient's daily activities.

Creating a Positive Atmosphere

A positive atmosphere can significantly impact the mood and well-being of both the care recipient and the caregiver.

Natural Light: Maximize natural light in the living space. Sunlight has been shown to improve mood and regulate sleep patterns.

Indoor Plants: Incorporate indoor plants to improve air quality and create a calming environment.

Decluttering: Keep the living space organized and free of clutter. A tidy environment can reduce stress and promote relaxation.

Animal Therapy: Animals can be very soothing and can provide comfort and companionship. At a care home where I train at, they hatched some duck eggs. Residents there and staff have marvelled at their progress, and they now live in the communal garden, giving great delight at their duck antics! Other homes or supported living environments have done this and it has been proven to benefit the people you are caring for.

Involving ME
Creating a supportive environment also benefits the caregiver by reducing stress and making caregiving tasks more manageable.

Caregiver Comfort: Ensure that the caregiver has a comfortable space to rest and recharge. This might include a cosy chair, a quiet corner, or access to relaxation tools like a massage chair or meditation apps.

Supportive Resources: Provide access to resources that support the caregiver's mental and physical health, such as support groups, counselling services, and educational materials.

Conclusion

Creating a supportive environment is a vital aspect of caregiving that enhances the quality of life for both the care recipient and the caregiver. By understanding the care recipient's needs, making physical and emotional adjustments, and utilizing technology and assistive devices, caregivers can create a space that promotes comfort, safety, and well-being. This approach not only benefits the care recipient but also reduces the caregiver's stress and improves their ability to provide effective care.

10.3 Encouraging Participation in Activities

Introduction

Encouraging participation in activities is crucial for maintaining the mental and physical health of care recipients. Engaging in meaningful activities can enhance cognitive function, reduce anxiety and depression, and improve the overall quality of life. This module explores strategies to encourage participation in activities that benefit both care recipients and caregivers.

1. Understanding the Importance of Activities

Activities play a vital role in the well-being of care recipients by providing structure, stimulation, and a sense of purpose.

- **Mental Stimulation:** Activities that challenge the brain, such as puzzles, reading, or learning new skills, can help maintain cognitive function and delay cognitive decline.
- **Physical Health**: Physical activities, even simple ones like walking or stretching, promote physical health, improve mobility, and reduce the risk of chronic diseases.
- **Emotional Well-being:** Engaging in enjoyable activities can boost mood, reduce stress, and provide a sense of accomplishment.

2. Tailoring Activities to Individual Preferences

To encourage participation, it's important to tailor activities to the care recipient's interests and abilities.

- **Personal Interests:** Identify activities that the care recipient enjoys or has enjoyed in the past. This could include hobbies like gardening, cooking, or playing a musical instrument.
- **Abilities and Limitations:** Consider the care recipient's physical and cognitive abilities when selecting activities. Adapt activities as needed to ensure they are manageable and enjoyable.

3. Creating a Routine for Activities

Incorporating activities into a daily routine can help make them a regular and anticipated part of the care recipient's day.

- **Daily Schedule:** Integrate a variety of activities into the daily schedule, balancing physical, mental, and social activities. Consistency helps establish a sense of routine and predictability.
- **Flexibility:** While routine is important, it's also essential to be flexible and adapt activities based on the care recipient's mood and energy levels.

4. Encouraging Social Interaction

Social activities can reduce feelings of isolation and loneliness, providing emotional support and enhancing the care recipient's well-being.

- **Group Activities:** Organize group activities, such as board games, book clubs, or social gatherings, to encourage interaction with others.
- **Family and Friends:** Encourage visits from family and friends and involve them in activities that the care recipient enjoys.

5. Exploring New Interests

Introducing new activities can stimulate curiosity and provide new avenues for enjoyment.

- **Trying New Hobbies:** Encourage the care recipient to try new hobbies or revisit old ones they may have enjoyed in the past. This could include painting, knitting, or playing a new game.
- **Community Programs:** Explore community programs and classes that offer opportunities for learning and social interaction. Many communities offer classes in art, music, fitness, and more

> **"Some activities can be designed to give caregivers a break. For example, if the care recipient enjoys watching a particular TV show or listening to an audiobook, this can provide some respite for the caregiver."**

6. Physical Activities

Physical activities are essential for maintaining health and mobility.

- **Simple Exercises:** Incorporate simple exercises like walking, stretching, or chair exercises into the daily routine. These activities can improve flexibility, strength, and balance.
- **Outdoor Activities:** Take advantage of outdoor activities, such as gardening, walking in the park, or birdwatching, to combine physical exercise with the benefits of being in nature.

7. Creative and Cognitive Activities

Engaging in creative and cognitive activities can provide mental stimulation and a sense of accomplishment.

- **Arts and Crafts:** Encourage participation in arts and crafts, such as painting, drawing, or knitting. These activities can be both relaxing and rewarding.
- **Puzzles and Games:** Provide puzzles, crosswords, and board games that challenge the mind and provide a fun way to spend time.

8. Adapting Activities for Different Conditions

Different health conditions may require specific adaptations to activities.

- **Dementia:** For individuals with dementia, choose activities that are simple, repetitive, and familiar. Activities like sorting objects, folding laundry, or looking through photo albums can be soothing and enjoyable.
- **Autism:** For individuals with autism, structure and predictability are key. Use visual aids to explain activities and ensure a calm and sensory-friendly environment.
- **Physical Disabilities:** Adapt activities to accommodate physical limitations. This might involve using assistive devices or modifying the activity to make it more accessible.

Conclusion

Encouraging participation in activities is a crucial aspect of caregiving that enhances the well-being of both the care recipient and the caregiver. By tailoring activities to individual preferences, creating a routine, and exploring new interests, caregivers can provide meaningful engagement that supports mental, physical, and emotional health. This approach not only enriches the lives of care recipients but also creates positive experiences and reduces stress for caregivers.

10.4
Thinking Outside The Box

Introduction

Caregiving often requires creativity and flexibility. Like actors adapting to different roles and audiences, caregivers must sometimes think outside the box to find effective solutions for their loved ones. In this module, we'll explore how innovative approaches can enhance caregiving, using real-life examples to illustrate the power of unconventional methods.

1. The Importance of Adaptability

Caregiving is not a one-size-fits-all endeavour. Each person is unique, with different needs, preferences, and responses. Being adaptable means being open to trying new things and willing to change tactics when something isn't working.

- **Personalized Approaches:** Tailor your caregiving methods to fit the individual. What works for one person may not work for another, so be ready to experiment with different strategies.
- **Flexibility:** Stay flexible in your approach. If a particular method isn't effective, don't be afraid to try something new.

2. Creativity in Caregiving

Creativity in caregiving can involve simple, yet imaginative changes to daily routines and interactions. These changes can lead to significant improvements in the well-being of the care recipient.

- **Engaging Activities:** Find activities that the care recipient enjoys and that stimulate their mind and body. This could be anything from arts and crafts to gardening or dancing.
- **Incorporating Interests:** Use the care recipient's interests to guide your activities. For example, if they love music, incorporate music into their daily routine.

Real-Life Example: The Power of Music

Consider the story of a caregiver who used music to reach a person with dementia who had become increasingly withdrawn and reluctant to get out of bed.

The Situation: *The care recipient had started doing less for themselves and was often reluctant to communicate. They would stay in bed for long periods and show little interest in daily activities.*

The Spark: *One day, the caregiver heard the care recipient singing a tune. Recognizing the potential in this moment, the caregiver decided to try something different.*

The Approach: *The caregiver ran into the room and started singing the tune, improvising new lyrics. This playful interaction was like a light switch in the care recipient's mind. They engaged in a "sing-off" with the caregiver, creating a lively and joyful atmosphere.*

The Result: *After a fun exchange, the caregiver sang, "Now would you like to get up and have some breakfast?" The care recipient sung back that they would. After two weeks of remaining in bed, they leapt out of bed, got dressed, and went to the dining room. This method became a regular part of their routine, transforming their mornings.*

3. Techniques to Consider

Different techniques can be employed to address various challenges in caregiving. Here are a few to inspire your creative thinking:

- **Role Play:** Sometimes, taking on a different persona can make routine tasks more engaging. For example, pretending to be a chef while preparing meals together can turn cooking into a fun activity.
- **Storytelling:** Use storytelling to engage the care recipient, especially if they enjoy certain genres or have favourite tales from their past. This can be particularly effective for individuals with dementia, as it taps into long-term memory.
- **Sensory Stimulation:** Engage multiple senses to create a stimulating environment. Use colours, textures, scents, and sounds to enhance the care recipient's experience.
- **Games and Challenges:** Introduce games or small challenges related to daily tasks. Turning tasks into a game can make them more enjoyable and less daunting.

4. Overcoming Resistance

When traditional methods fail, thinking outside the box can help overcome resistance and improve cooperation.

- **Changing the Narrative:** Reframe tasks to make them more appealing. For example, if the care recipient dislikes taking medication, turn it into a part of a "health hero" routine, where they earn badges or rewards for each dose taken.
- **Positive Reinforcement:** Use positive reinforcement to encourage participation. Celebrate small victories and milestones to build confidence and motivation.
- **Humour and Fun:** Inject humour and fun into caregiving tasks. A light-hearted approach can diffuse tension and make daily activities more enjoyable for both the caregiver and the care recipient.

Conclusion

Thinking outside the box in caregiving can lead to breakthroughs that significantly enhance the quality of life for both the care recipient and the caregiver. By being adaptable, creative, and open to new methods, caregivers can find innovative solutions to challenges and create a more engaging, supportive environment. Remember, caregiving is an art as much as it is a science, and sometimes, the most unexpected approaches yield the most rewarding results.

An Actor came singing.

In a quiet room, with curtains drawn tight,
Lay a lady lost, in the dim morning light.
Days she spent nestled in sheets of soft Gray,
Night blending into day, in the gentlest way.

Then came a morning, unexpected and bright,
With a budding actor stepping into her sight.
With a tune on his lips and a twinkle in his eye,
He sang to the lady, under the pale sky.

His voice like a lark, soared high and clear,
A melody sweet for her heart to hear.
"Rise and shine, oh sleeper, take my hand,"
He sang with a smile, his presence so grand.

Her toes tapped the rhythm, her heart felt the beat,
A dawning of joy as she moved her feet.
From the comfort of bed, she rose with a twirl,
Inspired by the song that made her world swirl.

Together they sang, a duet so bright,
Turning her gloom into glorious light.
For the actor had sung not just a tune,
But a call to life that made her bloom.

Now every morning, she greets the sun,
With a song in her heart, a new day begun.
For music had touched where nothing could reach,
A lesson in joy, that only love could teach.

CHAPTER 11

LEGAL & FINANCIAL CONSIDERATIONS

"Navigating legal and financial matters is like wrestling an octopus: just when you think you've got one tentacle under control, eight more come out of nowhere demanding signatures."

11.1
Understanding Caregiver Rights

Introduction

Caregivers play a crucial role in supporting loved ones, yet they often face numerous legal and financial challenges. Understanding caregiver rights is essential to ensure that caregivers are protected and supported. This module compares the caregiver rights in the United Kingdom, the United States, Canada, and Australia, highlighting key protections and benefits in each country. This can affect your mental health. In this chapter we will briefly explore this area, but it is always important to do additional research, depending which country you are from.

United Kingdom

In the United Kingdom, caregivers have specific rights and protections under the law. The Carers (Recognition and Services) Act 1995, the Carers and Disabled Children Act 2000, and the Care Act 2014 are primary legislative frameworks that provide these rights.

- **Carer's Assessment:** Caregivers are entitled to a carer's assessment to evaluate their needs. This assessment can result in support such as respite care, financial assistance, and training.

- **Financial Support:** Carer's Allowance is a financial benefit available to those who spend at least 35 hours a week caring for someone with substantial needs. Other financial supports include Carer's Credit and access to certain benefits and discounts.

- **Employment Rights:** The Employment Rights Act 1996 and the Work and Families Act 2006 grant caregivers the right to request flexible working arrangements and take time off for emergencies involving dependents.

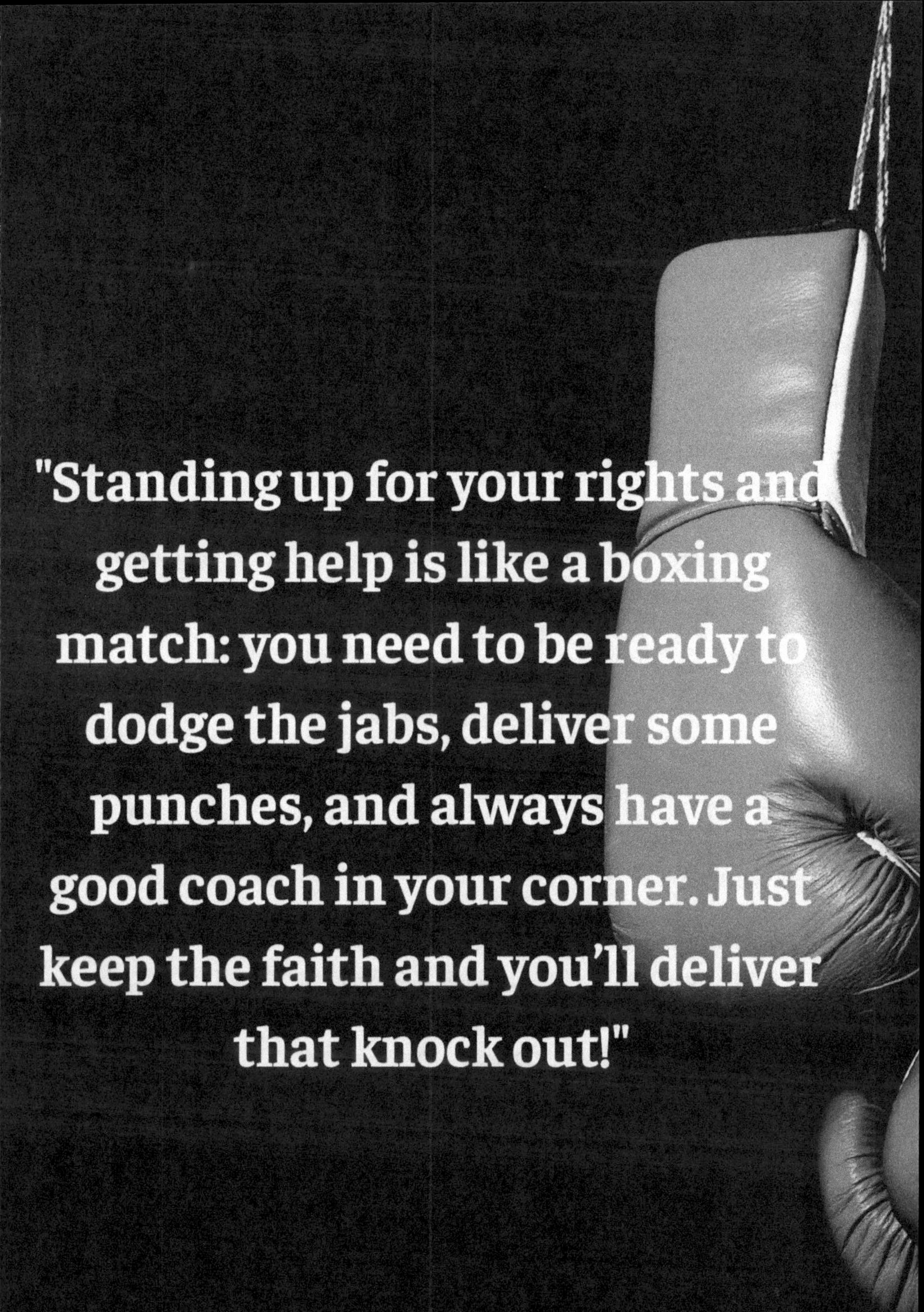

"Standing up for your rights and getting help is like a boxing match: you need to be ready to dodge the jabs, deliver some punches, and always have a good coach in your corner. Just keep the faith and you'll deliver that knock out!"

United States

In the United States, caregiver rights and supports are less standardized and vary widely by state. However, there are several federal provisions that offer protection and assistance.

- **Family and Medical Leave Act (FMLA):** Provides eligible employees with up to 12 weeks of unpaid leave per year to care for a family member with a serious health condition. During this time, their job is protected.

- **National Family Caregiver Support Program (NFCSP):** Offers grants to states to fund a range of support services for caregivers, including respite care, counseling, and training.

- **Medicaid Waivers:** Some states offer Medicaid waivers that provide financial assistance to family caregivers. The specifics of these programs vary by state.

Canada

In Canada, caregiver rights are supported through a combination of federal and provincial programs.

- **Employment Insurance (EI) Caregiving Benefits:** Provides temporary income support to those who take time off work to provide care or support to a critically ill or injured person or someone needing end-of-life care.

- **Compassionate Care Benefits:** Part of the EI program, this benefit provides up to 26 weeks of financial support for caregivers of family members who are gravely ill.

- **Provincial Programs:** Various provinces have additional programs. For example, Ontario offers the Ontario Caregiver Tax Credit, and British Columbia provides the BC Family Caregiver Recognition Act.

Australia

Australia has a robust framework to support caregivers, emphasizing both financial and emotional support.

- **Carer Payment:** A means-tested income support payment for caregivers who are unable to work full-time due to their caregiving responsibilities.

- **Carer Allowance:** A supplementary payment for caregivers who provide additional daily care to someone with a disability or medical condition.

- **National Disability Insurance Scheme (NDIS):** Provides support for Australians with a disability, including assistance for their caregivers.

- **Flexible Work Arrangements:** The Fair Work Act 2009 grants caregivers the right to request flexible working arrangements.

Comparative Analysis

While the specifics of caregiver rights vary across the United Kingdom, the United States, Canada, and Australia, there are common themes in the types of support available:

- **Financial Assistance:** All four countries provide some form of financial support to caregivers, whether through direct payments, allowances, or tax credits.

- **Job Protection:** Each country has provisions to protect the employment rights of caregivers, allowing them to take leave or request flexible working arrangements.

- **Support Services:** Access to respite care, training, and other support services is a key component of caregiver rights in each nation.

Conclusion

Understanding caregiver rights is essential for ensuring that caregivers are supported and protected. By comparing the legal and financial considerations in the United Kingdom, the United States, Canada, and Australia, caregivers can better navigate their roles and access the resources they need. This knowledge empowers caregivers to advocate for themselves and their loved ones, making their challenging roles more manageable and sustainable.

11.2
Managing Healthcare Costs

Managing healthcare costs is a significant concern for caregivers, as the financial burden of caring for a loved one can be substantial. This module will explore strategies for managing healthcare costs in the United Kingdom, the United States, Canada, and Australia. By understanding the available resources and planning effectively, caregivers can better navigate the financial challenges of their roles and reduce the burden on themselves.

United Kingdom

In the United Kingdom, the National Health Service (NHS) provides a range of healthcare services free at the point of use, which significantly reduces the burden of healthcare costs. However, there are still out-of-pocket expenses that caregivers need to manage.

- **NHS Services:** Most medical services, including hospital care, general practitioner visits, and specialist consultations, are covered by the NHS. However, there may be costs associated with prescriptions, dental care, and eye care.

- **Prescription Costs:** While some individuals are eligible for free prescriptions (e.g., those over 60, under 16, or with certain medical conditions), others may need to pay. Pre-payment certificates (PPCs) can help reduce these costs for those who need multiple prescriptions.

- **Local Authority Support:** Local authorities can provide financial assistance for home modifications, equipment, and personal care services. Care needs assessments are essential to determine eligibility.

- **Charitable Organizations:** Numerous charities offer grants and financial assistance for specific needs, such as mobility aids or respite care.

United States

In the United States, managing healthcare costs can be particularly challenging due to the fragmented and privatized healthcare system.

- **Health Insurance:** Having comprehensive health insurance is crucial. This includes understanding the benefits and limitations of private insurance plans, Medicare (for those over 65 or with certain disabilities), and Medicaid (for low-income individuals).

- **Medicaid Waivers:** Some states offer Medicaid waivers that provide additional support for home and community-based services, which can help reduce out-of-pocket expenses.

- **Out-of-Pocket Maximums:** Many insurance plans have out-of-pocket maximums that limit the amount individuals must pay in a year. Understanding these limits can help caregivers plan their finances.

- **Nonprofit Organizations:** Many nonprofits and charities offer financial assistance, particularly for specific conditions like cancer or Alzheimer's disease. Programs like the Patient Advocate Foundation can help with co-payments and medical bills.

Canada

In Canada, the healthcare system is publicly funded, providing universal coverage for medically necessary services. However, caregivers may still face significant costs for non-covered services.

- **Provincial Health Insurance:** Each province provides healthcare coverage for essential services, but there may be differences in what is covered. It's important to understand the specific benefits and limitations of your provincial plan.

- **Extended Health Benefits:** Many employers offer extended health benefits that cover additional services such as prescription drugs, physiotherapy, and mental health services. If these are not available through an employer, private insurance is an option.

- **Tax Credits and Deductions:** Caregivers can take advantage of various tax credits and deductions, such as the Disability Tax Credit (DTC) and the Medical Expense Tax Credit (METC).

- **Community Resources:** Programs like the Canada Caregiver Credit and provincial support services can provide additional financial assistance.

Australia

Australia's healthcare system combines public and private elements, offering various ways to manage healthcare costs.

- **Medicare:** Medicare provides free or subsidized access to many healthcare services. Understanding what is covered by Medicare is essential for managing costs.

- **Private Health Insurance:** Private health insurance can cover additional services not included in Medicare, such as private hospital care, dental, and optical services. The Australian Government provides rebates on private health insurance premiums.

- **Pharmaceutical Benefits Scheme (PBS):** The PBS helps reduce the cost of prescription medications. Additionally, the Safety Net program limits the amount individuals spend on medications in a calendar year.

- **Carer Payment and Carer Allowance:** Financial support is available for those providing substantial care. The Carer Payment is an income support benefit, while the Carer Allowance provides a supplementary payment.

List of Costs to Consider

When managing healthcare costs, caregivers should prepare for a range of potential expenses:

Medical Expenses: Costs for doctor visits, hospital stays, surgeries, and specialist consultations.

Prescriptions: Out-of-pocket costs for medications, even with insurance or government coverage.

Dental Care: Routine check-ups, cleanings, and more extensive procedures.

Vision Care: Eye exams, glasses, and contact lenses.

Specialist Equipment: Mobility aids, home modifications, and assistive devices.

Therapies: Physiotherapy, occupational therapy, and mental health counseling.

Home Care Services: Costs for professional caregivers or nursing services at home.

Transportation: Expenses for traveling to and from medical appointments.

Respite Care: Temporary relief services for caregivers, including short-term stays in care facilities.

Insurance Premiums: Monthly or annual payments for health, dental, and vision insurance.

General Strategies for Managing Healthcare Costs

Plan and Budget: Creating a detailed budget that includes all potential healthcare costs can help caregivers manage their finances effectively.

Explore All Options: Research all available resources, including government programs, charitable organizations, and insurance benefits.

Negotiate Medical Bills: In some countries, medical bills can be negotiated. Don't hesitate to discuss payment plans or reduced fees with healthcare providers.

Keep Accurate Records: Maintain detailed records of all medical expenses, insurance claims, and out-of-pocket payments. This can be crucial for tax purposes and applying for financial assistance.

Seek Professional Advice: Financial advisors and care coaches can provide valuable guidance on managing healthcare costs and planning for the future.

Conclusion

Managing healthcare costs is a critical aspect of caregiving that requires careful planning and awareness of available resources. By understanding the healthcare systems and financial supports in their respective countries, caregivers in the United Kingdom, the United States, Canada, and Australia can better navigate the financial challenges they face. Taking proactive steps to manage these costs will not only ease the financial burden but also improve the quality of care provided to loved ones. By preparing yourself as a caregiver, you reduce the burden on yourself and ensure that both you and your loved ones receive the necessary support.

11.3
Legal Resources and Support

Introduction

Caregiving comes with a host of legal responsibilities and considerations. Navigating the legal landscape can be challenging, but understanding the available resources and support can make this process more manageable. In this module, we will explore legal resources and support available to caregivers in the United Kingdom, the United States, Canada, and Australia. This information will empower you to make informed decisions and ensure that you and your loved ones are protected. Further information can be found at the end of this eBook.

United Kingdom

In the UK, caregivers have access to various legal resources and support systems designed to help them navigate the complexities of caregiving.

- **Legal Aid:** Legal Aid provides financial assistance for legal representation and advice. It can cover issues like power of attorney, wills, and disputes regarding care.

- **Citizens Advice Bureau:** This organization offers free, confidential advice on legal and financial matters, including housing, benefits, and employment rights.

- **Solicitors for the Elderly:** A national organization of lawyers specializing in legal issues affecting older people and their caregivers. They can provide guidance on estate planning, lasting power of attorney, and care home contracts.

- **Court of Protection:** This court deals with cases involving people who lack the mental capacity to make their own decisions. It can appoint deputies to make decisions on behalf of a loved one.

United States

In the US, there are numerous legal resources available to caregivers to help them manage their responsibilities effectively.

- **Elder Law Attorneys:** These lawyers specialize in issues affecting the elderly, including estate planning, Medicaid planning, and guardianship. They can provide valuable guidance on legal matters specific to caregiving.

- **Legal Services Corporation:** A federally funded organization that provides civil legal aid to low-income Americans. They offer help with issues like healthcare access, public benefits, and housing.

- **National Academy of Elder Law Attorneys (NAELA):** This organization consists of attorneys specializing in elder law. They provide resources and referrals to qualified lawyers.

- **Area Agencies on Aging (AAA):** These agencies offer legal assistance programs that can help with issues like powers of attorney, advance directives, and consumer protection.

Canada

Canadian caregivers have access to various legal resources and support systems designed to assist them in their roles.

- **Legal Aid Services:** Each province and territory in Canada offers legal aid services to those who qualify financially. These services can assist with matters like estate planning, guardianship, and elder abuse.

- **Public Guardian and Trustee (PGT):** The PGT provides services to protect the legal rights of those who cannot manage their own affairs. They can help with managing finances, personal care, and legal decisions.

- **Community Legal Clinics:** These clinics offer free legal advice and representation to low-income individuals on a variety of issues, including housing, social assistance, and elder law.

- **Canadian Network for the Prevention of Elder Abuse (CNPEA):** This organization provides resources and information on legal issues related to elder abuse and the rights of older adults.

Australia

In Australia, caregivers can access a range of legal resources to help them navigate the complexities of caregiving.

- **Legal Aid Commissions:** Each state and territory has a legal aid commission that provides free or low-cost legal services to those who qualify. They can help with issues like guardianship, enduring power of attorney, and elder abuse.

- **Public Trustee Offices:** These offices offer services to manage the financial and legal affairs of those who cannot do so themselves. They provide assistance with estate planning, wills, and trusts.

- **Elder Law Solicitors:** Lawyers specializing in elder law can provide advice on a wide range of issues, including aged care agreements, retirement village contracts, and estate disputes.

- **Seniors Rights Service:** This organization offers free legal advice, advocacy, and education to older Australians. They can assist with issues related to aged care, retirement villages, and elder abuse.

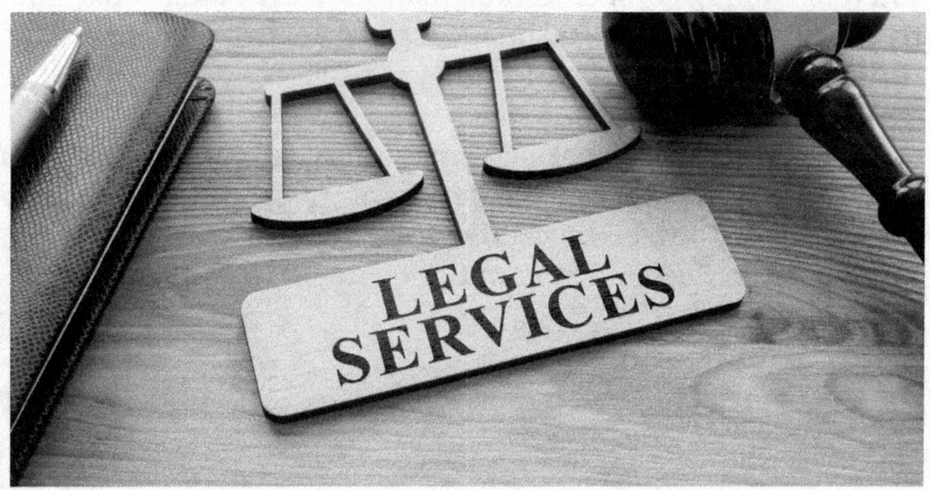

Additional Legal Considerations

Caregivers should also be aware of specific legal documents and considerations that can significantly impact their caregiving journey:

Power of Attorney: A legal document that allows a caregiver to make financial and legal decisions on behalf of a loved one. It's crucial to establish this early to ensure that there are no disruptions in care.

Advance Directives: These documents specify a person's wishes regarding medical treatment in the event they become unable to communicate those wishes themselves. They can include living wills and healthcare proxies.

Guardianship and Conservatorship: Legal processes to appoint someone to make decisions on behalf of an incapacitated individual. This can be a lengthy and complex process, so it's essential to understand the requirements and implications.

Estate Planning: Proper estate planning, including wills and trusts, ensures that a loved one's assets are distributed according to their wishes and can help avoid legal disputes.

Care Agreements: Formal agreements between caregivers and care recipients outlining the terms of care, including duties, compensation, and expectations. This can help prevent misunderstandings and conflicts.

Conclusion

Navigating the legal aspects of caregiving can be daunting, but there are numerous resources and supports available to help caregivers manage these responsibilities. By understanding the legal landscape and accessing the appropriate services, caregivers can protect themselves and their loved ones, ensuring a smoother and more secure caregiving journey. For more detailed information on specific legal resources and support available in your country, please refer to the appendix at the end of this eBook.

When In Rome.

In ancient Rome, a chancellor named Brice,
Had a job that was anything but nice.
To care for Caesar and fund his grand state,
While minding his own, a modest estate.

"Caesar needs gold for a new marble throne,
And fountains and feasts," Brice did bemoan.
"Yet my small villa, with its leaky roof,
Demands attention, and that's the truth!"

Brice juggled the books with a frown and a sigh,
"How to keep Caesar happy and my chickens dry?"
He taxed all the sandals and levied the togas,
But still found his funds just too little and bogus.

One day he declared, "I've had quite enough!
Caring for Caesar is really quite tough!
I'll host a grand circus, and make people pay,
To see gladiators and lions at play!"

The circus was packed, and gold filled his purse,
Brice felt his worries beginning to disperse.
"Now Caesar gets statues, and I'll fix my home,
At last, a solution for all of Rome!"

With Caesar content and his villa repaired,
Brice laughed at the chaos he'd so deftly spared.
For though it was tough, with humour and cheer,
He'd managed to balance his dual careers.

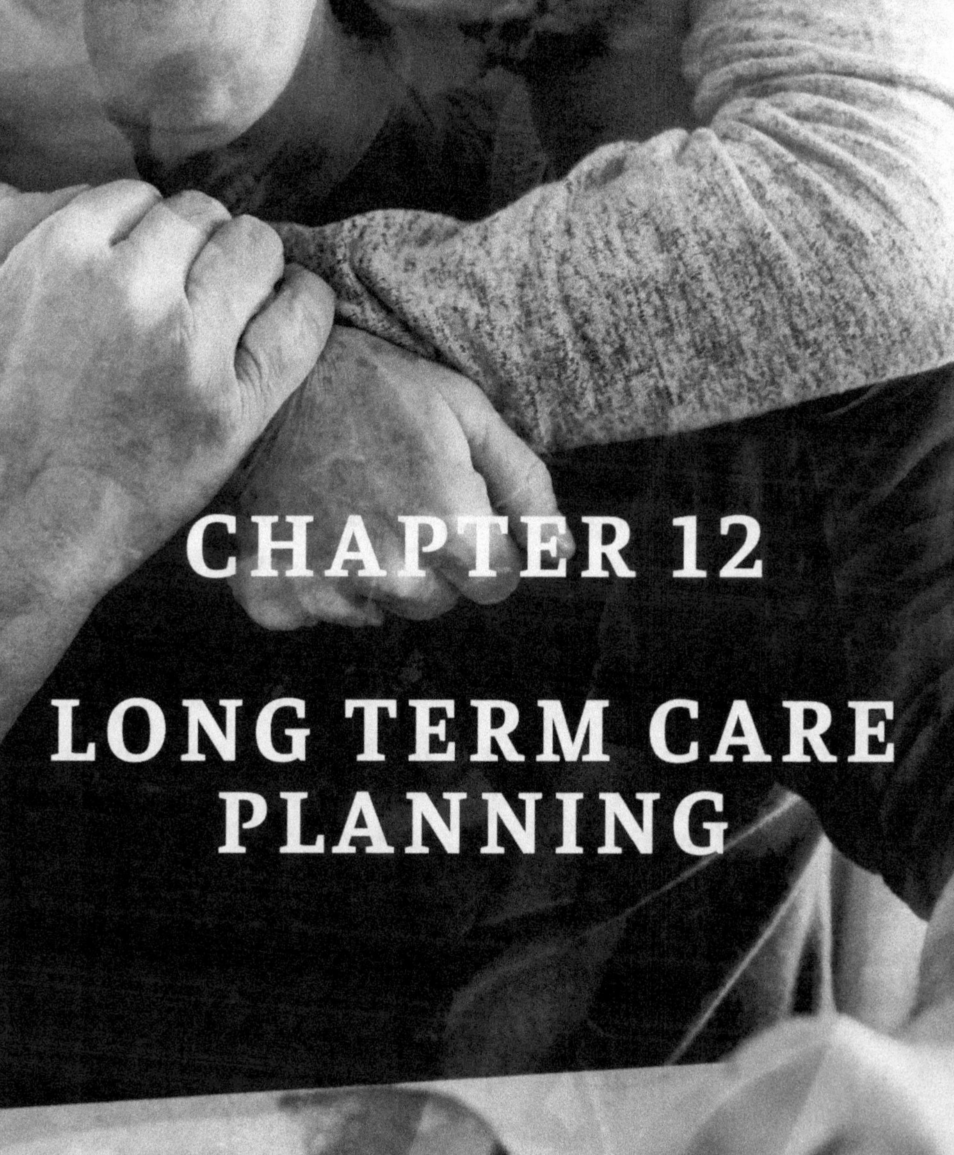

"Long-term care planning is like assembling IKEA furniture: it seems overwhelming at first, the instructions are confusing, and you'll probably need an extra set of hands, but in the end, it's worth it to avoid a wobbly future."

12.1
Planning For The Future

Introduction

Caring for someone with a variety of conditions including dementia, cerebral palsy, MS or severe special needs can take over your life, especially as you start to witness changes in the person you care for. Some changes are positive, like small victories in their progress, while others might be challenging, such as the worsening of certain symptoms. You've likely experienced both good and bad times, from moments of joy when they achieve a milestone to times of frustration and exhaustion when things don't go as planned. Despite the hardships, a special bond often forms, grounded in trust, empathy, and mutual reliance. This bond can be a source of strength, providing emotional support and a deep sense of connection that makes the caregiving journey worthwhile.

As a carer, self-care is essential, and part of self-care involves planning for the future. Caring for a loved one is a journey that often evolves and changes over time. Recognizing the need for professional help or considering supported living or care home environments can be daunting and emotionally taxing. Many carers experience feelings of guilt and a sense of failure when these options become necessary. However, acknowledging these feelings and understanding the importance of preparing for future care needs is crucial in providing the best support for your loved one and maintaining your own well-being. Proactively seeking out resources, support groups, and professional advice can help ease the transition, ensuring that your loved one continues to receive high-quality care while you maintain your health and balance.

Whilst you may feel that you have a duty of care to the person you are supporting, you also have a duty of care to yourself. Some people ignore this but it is essential you do not.

The Importance of Long-term Care Planning

Long-term care planning involves making arrangements for the ongoing support and care of your loved one as their needs change. This planning ensures that they receive appropriate care when you are no longer able to provide it yourself. By thinking ahead, you can avoid crises and ensure a smoother transition when the time comes to seek professional help or consider alternative living arrangements.

Key Aspects of Long-term Care Planning:

- Assessing Current and Future Needs

- Evaluate your loved one's current health status and care needs.

- Consider potential future needs based on their medical condition and prognosis.

- Recognize your own limitations and the possibility that your ability to provide care may change over time.

Involving Your Loved One

- Involve your loved one in discussions about their future care whenever possible.

- Respect their preferences and consider their wishes in the decision-making process.

- Open and honest communication can help reduce anxiety and ensure that their voice is heard.

Personal Note: I remember when my Grandfather passed. Even though I was young, I had the impression that my Grandmother had no choices and was sent to a care home. As I have got older, I have heard this a lot. INVOLVE THEM WHEN EVER YOU CAN! THEY ARE A PERSON!

Exploring Care Options

- Research various care options, including in-home care services, supported living arrangements, and care homes.

- Understand the benefits and drawbacks of each option to make an informed decision.

- Consider factors such as cost, location, quality of care, and the specific needs of your loved one.

Financial Planning

- Assess the financial implications of different care options.

- Explore funding sources such as insurance, government programs, and personal savings.

- Seek advice from financial advisors or elder care planners to manage costs effectively.

Legal Considerations

- Ensure that legal documents such as wills, powers of attorney, and advance directives are in place.

- Consult with legal professionals to understand the legal aspects of long-term care planning.

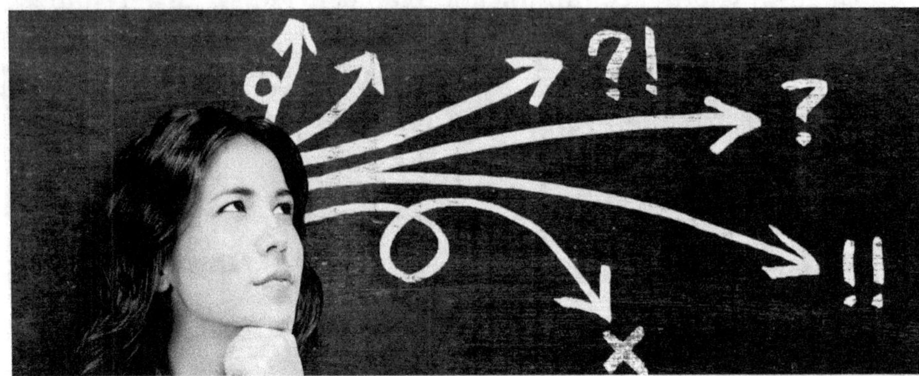

Addressing Emotional Challenges

The transition to professional care or a care home can be emotionally challenging for both the carer and the person being cared for. Feelings of guilt, failure, and loss are common, but it's essential to address these emotions constructively.

- Managing Guilt and a Sense of Failure:

- Acknowledge Your Emotions

- Recognize that feelings of guilt and failure are natural.

- Accept that you are doing your best and that seeking help is not a sign of inadequacy.

Seek Support

- Connect with other carers who have gone through similar experiences.

- Join support groups to share your feelings and gain perspective.

- Consider counselling or therapy to process your emotions.

Focus on the Positives

- Remind yourself of the positive impact you have had on your loved one's life.

- Recognize that professional care can provide specialized support that you may not be able to offer.

Reframe Your Perspective

- Understand that seeking professional help is a responsible and caring decision.

- Viewing this transition as a step towards ensuring the best possible care for your loved one can help alleviate feelings of guilt.

Examples and Scenarios

Example 1

Involving Your Loved One in Decision-Making

Sarah has been caring for her mother, who has Alzheimer's disease, for several years. As her mother's condition progresses, Sarah realizes that her mother needs more specialized care than she can provide at home.

Sarah sits down with her mother and has a gentle conversation about the possibility of moving to a care home that specializes in dementia care.

Despite her mother's limited ability to fully understand the situation, Sarah involves her in the process by visiting care homes together and discussing her preferences for a living environment.

This approach helps Sarah's mother feel valued and respected, easing the transition.

Examples and Scenarios

Example 2

Managing Guilt and Seeking Support

John has been caring for his wife, who has advanced multiple sclerosis, at home. As her condition worsens, John struggles with the physical and emotional demands of caregiving.

He feels guilty at the thought of moving her to a care home. John joins a local support group for carers, where he meets others who have faced similar decisions. Hearing their stories and sharing his own experiences helps John realize that seeking professional care is not a failure but a necessary step to ensure his wife's well-being and his own health.

With the support of the group, John finds the strength to make the decision and transition his wife to a care home.

Examples and Scenarios

Example 3

Exploring Care Options and Financial Planning

Emma's father has Parkinson's disease and requires increasing levels of care. Emma begins to explore various care options, including in-home care services and assisted living facilities.

She consults with a financial advisor to understand the costs and funding sources available. Together, they create a financial plan that includes long-term care insurance, personal savings, and potential government assistance.

By planning ahead, Emma ensures that her father will receive the necessary care without compromising their financial stability.

Conclusion: Hope for the Future

Long-term care planning is an essential aspect of being a carer. By preparing for the future, involving your loved one in decision-making, and addressing emotional challenges, you can ensure the best possible care for your loved one while maintaining your own well-being.

Remember that seeking professional help is a responsible and caring choice, not a sign of failure. With thoughtful planning and support, you can navigate the complexities of long-term care and find hope for the future.

Key Takeaways:

- Assess current and future care needs.
- Involve your loved one in planning whenever possible.
- Explore various care options and understand their implications.
- Address emotional challenges such as guilt and a sense of failure.
- Seek support from other carers and professionals.
- Plan financially and legally to ensure long-term stability.

By following these steps, you can create a comprehensive long-term care plan that provides peace of mind for you and your loved one. Preparing for the future is an act of love and responsibility, ensuring that your loved one receives the best possible care while allowing you to continue providing support in a sustainable way.

12.2
If You Need to Put Someone in Care

The decision to place a loved one in a care home is one of the most difficult and emotionally charged choices a carer can face. Even after dedicating yourself to their care, there may come a time when professional help is necessary. It's important to understand that care homes have their own methods and routines, which may differ from your approach. Additionally, the progression of your loved one's condition may cause them to behave in ways that seem unfamiliar or alien. Understanding these factors can help manage expectations and reduce unnecessary stress.

The Reality of Transitioning to a Care Home

When a loved one moves into a care home, it can be a time of significant adjustment for both of you. It's natural to feel a sense of loss or even guilt, but it's important to remember that this step is taken with their best interests in mind.

Understanding Different Approaches

Care homes have established protocols and routines designed to provide the best care possible for their residents. These methods may differ from how you managed care at home, but they are based on professional standards and experience.

Structured Environment

- Care homes provide a structured environment with routines that help residents feel secure.

- Activities are scheduled to promote social interaction and mental stimulation.

Specialized Staff

- Trained professionals, including nurses, therapists, and care assistants, offer specialized care.

- Staff members are equipped to handle complex medical and behavioural issues.

Community Setting

Living in a community with other residents can provide social benefits and reduce feelings of isolation.

- Shared activities and communal dining foster a sense of belonging.

Progression of the Condition

As your loved one's condition advances, their behaviour and needs may change significantly. Many people often blame or criticise the care home as the progression of the condition. These changes can be distressing but understanding them can help you adjust.

Cognitive Decline

Conditions like dementia can lead to significant changes in behaviour and personality.

- Your loved one may not always recognize you or respond as they once did.

Physical Health

Progressive conditions can lead to decreased mobility and increased dependence on others for daily activities.

- Professional caregivers are trained to manage these changes effectively.

Emotional Well-being

Emotional fluctuations are common as individuals adjust to their new environment.

- Care homes provide support to help residents cope with these changes.

Managing Expectations and Emotions

Transitioning a loved one into a care home can be emotionally challenging. It's essential to manage expectations and understand that care homes strive to provide the best possible care.

Common Emotional Responses

Guilt

- Feeling guilty is a common reaction, but it's important to remember that you are making the best decision for your loved one's well-being.

- Acknowledge your feelings and seek support from friends, family, or support groups.

Blame

- It's easy to blame the care home for any perceived shortcomings, but understanding their methods can help alleviate these feelings.

- Communicate openly with the care home staff to address any concerns.

Loss

- The sense of loss when your loved one moves into a care home is profound.

- Focus on the positive aspects of their new environment, such as increased social interaction and professional care.

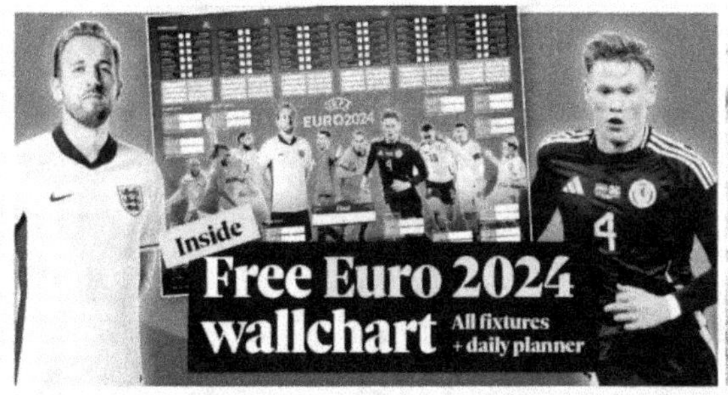

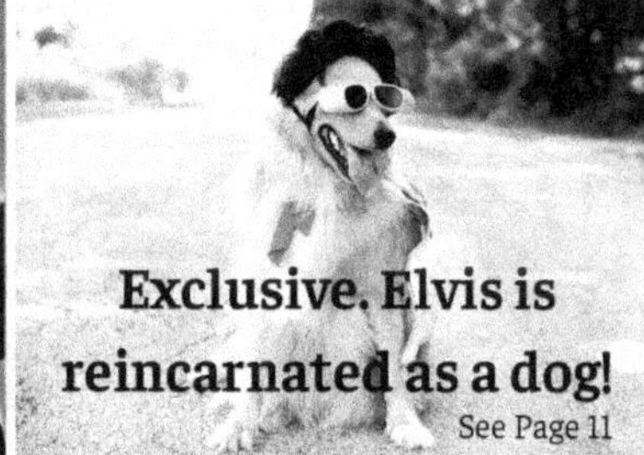

Exclusive. Elvis is reincarnated as a dog!
See Page 11

DAILY NEWS

Delivering the News Every Day   Sunday 9th June 2024

AMAZING CARE GIVEN ONCE AGAIN TO BETTY BY HER CARER ! ! !

- **PERSON CENTRED CARE**
- **CHOICES**
- **DIGNITY**

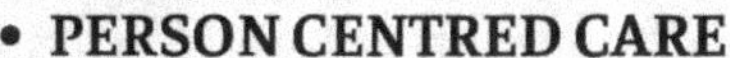

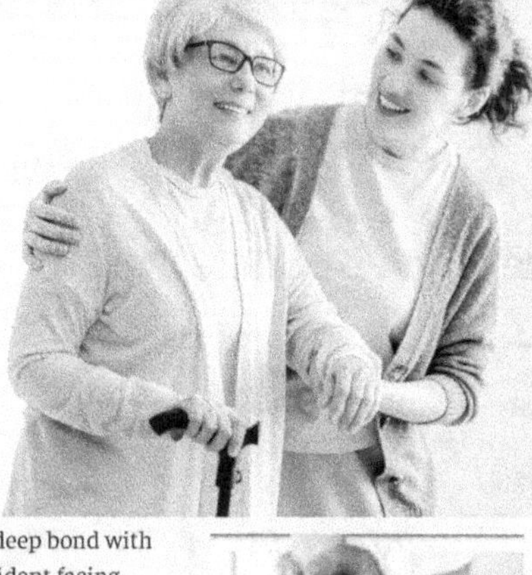

Breaking News: Exceptional Care Reported at We Care Home by Iva Carer for Resident Betty Lovedone

In a heartwarming development, We Care Home has become the center of attention due to the extraordinary care provided by Iva Carer to resident Betty Lovedone. This story of dedication and compassion is rapidly gaining recognition and admiration. Unwavering Commitment and Personalized Care. Iva Carer has been praised for her empathetic and detailed approach to caregiving.

She has developed a deep bond with Betty Lovedone, a resident facing significant health challenges. Iva's commitment goes beyond basic duties, as she takes the time to understand Betty's history and preferences, ensuring she feels valued and understood.

Iva's innovative methods, including personalized music therapy sessions, have shown remarkable results in enhancing Betty's mood and cognitive function. This tailored approach has significantly improved

Cont. page 2

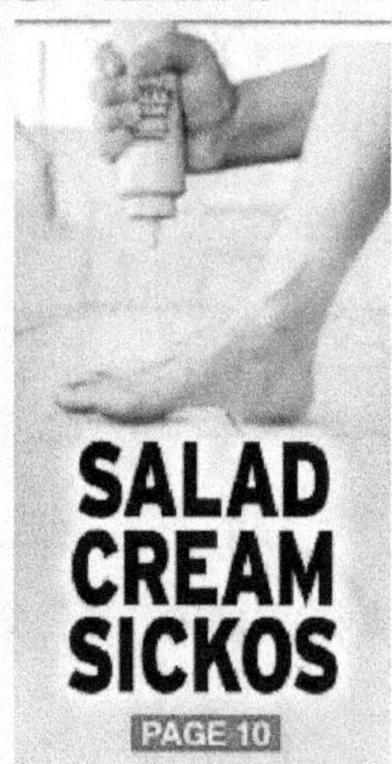

Trusting the Care Home

Care homes are dedicated to providing quality care for their residents. We always hear the bad stories. These are in the minority. Would the newspapers put on their front page "Amazing care done by carers again today!" If they did, it would be on the front page every day because there is some amazing care being done in care homes". Trusting their expertise and understanding their approach can help ease the transition.

Reasons Behind Their Methods

Safety and Health

- Care homes implement routines and protocols to ensure the safety and health of all residents.

- These measures may include scheduled medication times, dietary plans, and specific hygiene practices.

Individualized Care Plans

- Each resident has an individualized care plan tailored to their specific needs.

- Staff members are trained to follow these plans and adapt as necessary.

Professional Standards

- Care homes adhere to regulatory standards and best practices in the industry.

- Regular training and assessments ensure that staff provide high-quality care. These include manual handling (I call it moving and assisting as we don't manually handle people!), first aid, fire safety, Safeguarding and many more.

Communication is Key

Open Dialogue

Maintain an open line of communication with the care home staff.

Discuss any concerns or questions you have about your loved one's care.

Visiting and Participating

Regular visits can help you stay connected with your loved one and their care routine.

Participate in care home events and activities to understand their environment better.

Feedback and Collaboration

Provide feedback to the care home staff and collaborate on any adjustments needed.

Positive communication fosters a supportive relationship between you and the caregivers.

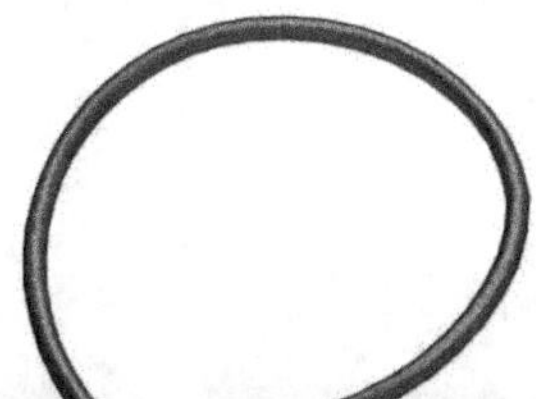

Examples and Scenarios

Example 1

Understanding Different Care Approaches

Maria moved her father, who has advanced Parkinson's disease, into a care home. Initially, she was upset to see that the staff handled his daily routine differently than she did at home. However, after discussing with the care home's manager, Maria learned that the structured routine was designed to provide stability and reduce anxiety for residents.

Understanding this helped her appreciate the professional approach and feel more at ease.

Examples and Scenarios

Example 2

Managing Guilt and Building Trust

Tom felt overwhelming guilt after placing his wife, who has Alzheimer's, into a care home. He blamed himself for not being able to care for her at home anymore. By joining a support group, Tom connected with other carers who had faced similar decisions. He also started having regular meetings with the care home staff to stay informed about his wife's care plan.

Over time, Tom learned to trust the caregivers and saw how their expertise benefited his wife.

Examples and Scenarios

Example 3

Communicating and Collaborating

Linda was concerned when she noticed her mother's dietary routine had changed after moving to a care home. She scheduled a meeting with the care home's nutritionist and learned that the new diet was designed to address her mother's specific health needs. Linda provided feedback on her mother's food preferences, and the nutritionist adjusted the menu accordingly.

This collaboration improved her mother's well-being and eased Linda's concerns.

So Many Success Stories

There are countless success stories of individuals thriving in care homes, though these stories often go unheard. Consider the story of Mark, a young man diagnosed with learning difficulties, autism, and a rare form of epilepsy. When living with his parents, Mark frequently displayed challenging behaviours that escalated to crises, often resulting in aggression towards his parents. His family, reluctantly seeking help, placed him into a supported living environment.

Initially, the transition was difficult, but over time, Mark began to settle. The structured environment and dedicated 1:1 care provided by trained professionals allowed Mark to thrive. His challenging behaviours subsided significantly as he adjusted to his new surroundings. Where Mark once required the constant presence of at least two carers, he now benefits from the support of just one carer.

Mark enjoys an active and fulfilling life, engaging in various activities and building meaningful relationships. His parents visit regularly, cherishing their time together and witnessing the positive changes in Mark's well-being.

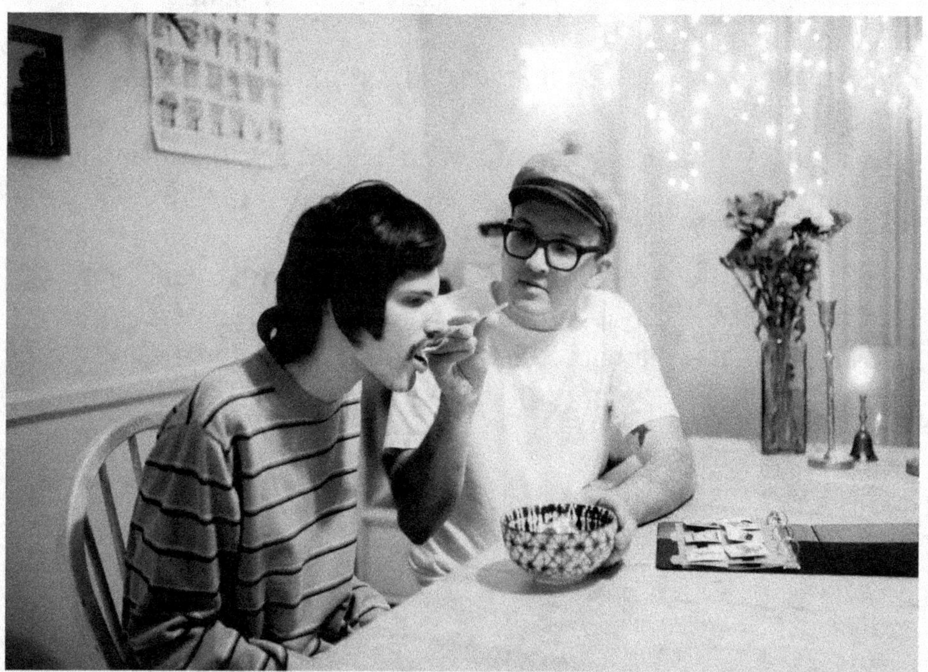

Conclusion: Embracing the Transition

Placing a loved one in a care home is a significant and often emotional decision. Understanding that care homes have their own methods, recognizing the progression of your loved one's condition, and managing your expectations can help ease the transition. Trust that care homes are committed to providing quality care and maintaining open communication with the staff to address any concerns.

Key Takeaways:

- Care homes have structured routines and specialized staff to provide the best care.
- The progression of your loved one's condition may lead to changes that seem unfamiliar.
- Manage emotional responses such as guilt and blame constructively.
- Trust the care home's methods and communicate openly with the staff.
- Regular visits and participation can help you stay connected and informed.

By embracing these principles, you can ensure that your loved one receives the necessary care while maintaining your peace of mind. Remember that seeking professional help is a responsible and caring decision that reflects your commitment to your loved one's well-being.

12.3
Advanced Care Directives

Understanding Advanced Care Directives
Advanced care directives (ACDs) are legal documents that outline a person's preferences for medical treatment and care in situations where they may no longer be able to communicate their decisions. These directives provide critical guidance to healthcare providers and loved ones, ensuring that a person's wishes are respected and followed during times of serious illness or incapacity. For carers, understanding and implementing ACDs is an essential aspect of long-term care planning.

The Importance of Advanced Care Directives

- Respecting Autonomy

- Honouring Preferences:

- ACDs ensure that a person's values, beliefs, and preferences for medical treatment are respected.

- They provide clear instructions on what types of care and interventions are acceptable or unacceptable to the individual.

Empowering Individuals:
By creating ACDs, individuals can make proactive decisions about their future healthcare.

This empowerment can provide peace of mind, knowing that their wishes will be honoured even if they cannot communicate them.

Reducing Stress and Uncertainty

Clarity for Carers and Families:
- ACDs remove ambiguity, making it easier for carers and family members to make decisions during stressful and emotional times.

- They prevent conflicts and disagreements among family members about the best course of action.

Guidance for Healthcare Providers:
Healthcare professionals rely on ACDs to provide care that aligns with the patient's wishes.

These directives ensure that medical interventions are consistent with the individual's values and preferences.

Supporting Ethical and Legal Standards

Legal Protection:
- ACDs provide legal documentation that healthcare providers must follow, protecting the individual's rights.

- They help avoid legal disputes over the appropriateness of medical treatments and interventions.

Ethical Decision-Making:
- ACDs support ethical medical practices by ensuring that treatment aligns with the patient's expressed wishes.

- They promote patient-centred care and respect for individual autonomy.

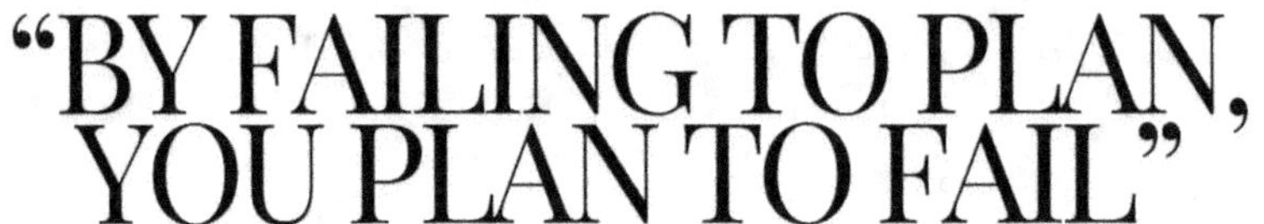

Types of Advanced Care Directives

Living Wills
Purpose and Scope: A living will outline specific medical treatments and interventions that an individual wishes to receive or avoid. It typically addresses scenarios such as life support, resuscitation, and end-of-life care.

Implementation: Living wills become effective when the individual is incapacitated and unable to communicate their decisions. Healthcare providers use this document to guide treatment decisions in accordance with the individual's preferences.

Durable Power of Attorney for Healthcare
Role and Responsibilities: This document designates a trusted person (agent or proxy) to make healthcare decisions on behalf of the individual. The appointed agent has the authority to make decisions in situations not explicitly covered by the living will.

Choosing an Agent: The chosen agent should be someone who understands the individual's values and preferences and is willing to advocate on their behalf. It's essential to have open discussions with the designated agent about the individual's wishes and expectations.

Do Not Resuscitate (DNR) Orders
Definition and Purpose: A DNR order specifies that an individual does not want to receive cardiopulmonary resuscitation (CPR) if their heart stops or they stop breathing. This order is typically used for individuals with serious, terminal, or life-limiting conditions.

Communication with Healthcare Providers: DNR orders should be clearly communicated to all healthcare providers and included in the individual's medical records. Wearing a medical alert bracelet or carrying a DNR card can help ensure that this directive is followed in emergencies.

How Advanced Care Directives Support Carers

Providing Guidance and Direction
Clear Instructions: ACDs offer clear, written instructions that carers can follow, reducing uncertainty and anxiety about making medical decisions. They ensure that the carer's actions are aligned with the individual's wishes.

Decision-Making Support: Having ACDs in place provides carers with the authority and confidence to advocate for the individual's preferences. They serve as a reference point during difficult conversations with healthcare providers and family members.

Reducing Emotional Burden
Alleviating Guilt and Stress: Knowing that they are following the individual's wishes can help carers feel more at ease with their decisions. ACDs reduce the emotional burden of second-guessing or questioning whether they are making the right choices.

Facilitating Communication: ACDs encourage open discussions between carers, the individual, and healthcare providers about care preferences. These conversations can strengthen the carer's understanding of the individual's values and improve the quality of care.

Legal and Ethical Assurance
Legal Protection: ACDs provide legal backing for the carer's decisions, reducing the risk of disputes or challenges from other family members. They ensure that the individual's rights are protected, and their wishes are legally upheld.

Ethical Confidence: Carers can be confident that they are making ethically sound decisions based on the individual's expressed wishes. ACDs promote respect for the individual's autonomy and dignity.

Creating and Implementing Advanced Care Directives

Steps to Create Advanced Care Directives
Initiate the Conversation: Discuss the importance of ACDs with your loved one and encourage them to express their wishes. Use open-ended questions to explore their values, beliefs, and preferences for medical care.

Consult Healthcare Professionals: Seek advice from doctors, nurses, or elder care planners to understand the medical implications of various directives. Ensure that the ACDs are medically feasible and accurately reflect the individual's wishes.

Draft the Documents: Work with legal professionals to draft the necessary ACDs, including living wills, durable power of attorney for healthcare, and DNR orders.Ensure that the documents are clear, comprehensive, and legally valid.

Review and Revise: Regularly review the ACDs with your loved one to ensure that they remain up-to-date and reflect any changes in their preferences or medical condition. Make necessary revisions and revalidate the documents as needed.

Implementing Advanced Care Directives
Distribute Copies: Provide copies of the ACDs to all relevant parties, including healthcare providers, the designated agent, and family members. Keep a copy in an easily accessible location and ensure that the individual carries a copy with them.

Communicate Clearly: Inform all healthcare providers about the existence of the ACDs and ensure they are included in the individual's medical records. Clearly communicate any changes or updates to the directives promptly.

Advocate and Enforce: As a carer, advocate for the individual's wishes and ensure that the ACDs are respected and followed. Address any discrepancies or concerns with healthcare providers immediately to ensure compliance with the directives.

Conclusion: Empowering Care Through Advanced Care Directives

Advanced care directives are a crucial component of long-term care planning, providing clear guidance and legal assurance for carers and healthcare providers. By respecting the individual's wishes, reducing emotional burdens, and ensuring ethical and legal standards, ACDs empower carers to provide the best possible care. Initiating conversations, creating, and implementing these directives are essential steps in supporting your loved one's autonomy and dignity, ensuring that their preferences are honoured even in challenging circumstances.

12.4
Hospice and Palliative Care

Understanding Hospice and Palliative Care

Reaching the stage where hospice and palliative care become necessary can be a difficult and emotional time for both the carer and the loved one. However, it's important to understand that these services are designed to provide comfort, dignity, and support during the final stages of life. Embracing hospice and palliative care means prioritizing quality of life, ensuring that your loved one experiences a peaceful and dignified journey.

What Are Hospice and Palliative Care?

Hospice Care

End-of-Life Focus: Hospice care is intended for individuals who are nearing the end of life, typically with a prognosis of six months or less if the illness follows its expected course. The focus is on comfort rather than curative treatments, emphasizing pain management and emotional support.

Holistic Approach: Hospice care addresses the physical, emotional, spiritual, and social needs of the patient and their family. Care is provided by a team of healthcare professionals, including doctors, nurses, social workers, and chaplains.

Setting and Services: Hospice care can be provided at home, in a hospice facility, or within a hospital or nursing home. Services include pain and symptom management, counselling, respite care for family members, and bereavement support.

As a trainer and coach I have never seen such kindness than carers in Hospice Care

Palliative Care
Symptom Management: Palliative care focuses on relieving symptoms and improving quality of life for individuals with serious illnesses, regardless of the stage or prognosis. It can be provided alongside curative treatments or as a standalone approach.

Comprehensive Care: Palliative care teams work to address physical discomfort, as well as emotional, social, and spiritual concerns. The goal is to enhance comfort and support the patient and their family through all stages of the illness.

Flexible and Individualized: Palliative care is tailored to the individual's needs and preferences, evolving as their condition changes. It can be delivered in various settings, including hospitals, outpatient clinics, and at home.

The Importance of Hospice and Palliative Care

Ensuring Dignity and Comfort
Respecting Wishes: Hospice and palliative care prioritize the patient's wishes, ensuring that their end-of-life experience aligns with their values and preferences. This approach allows individuals to maintain control and dignity during their final days.

Managing Pain and Symptoms: Expert pain management and symptom relief are central to hospice and palliative care, ensuring that patients remain as comfortable as possible. This alleviates suffering and enhances the quality of life for both the patient and their family.

Providing Emotional and Spiritual Support: Emotional and spiritual care is a key component, helping patients and their families navigate the complex emotions associated with end-of-life. Support services include counselling, chaplain visits, and grief support for loved ones. At the end, even non-believers sometimes want spiritual support.

Supporting the Family

Respite Care: Hospice provides respite care, allowing primary carers to take a break and recharge while knowing their loved one is in good hands. This helps prevent caregiver burnout and maintains the carer's well-being.

Bereavement Support: After the loss of a loved one, hospice offers bereavement support to help families cope with grief and loss. Services may include counselling, support groups, and resources for navigating the grieving process.

Education and Guidance: Hospice and palliative care teams provide education on what to expect during the end-of-life process, empowering families with knowledge and preparation. This guidance helps families feel more in control and less anxious about the unknown.

Embracing Hospice and Palliative Care

Making the Decision

Recognizing the Need: It's important to recognize when curative treatments are no longer effective and the focus should shift to comfort and quality of life. Honest conversations with healthcare providers can help determine the appropriate time to transition to hospice or palliative care.

Discussing Preferences: Engage in open discussions with your loved one about their end-of-life wishes and preferences. Document these preferences through advanced care directives to ensure they are honoured.

Seeking Support: Reach out to hospice and palliative care services for information and support in making the transition. These professionals can provide valuable insights and help ease the process.

Examples and Scenarios

Example 1

Providing Comfort and Peace

Sarah's father, James, was diagnosed with advanced cancer. As his condition worsened, curative treatments were no longer effective, and his pain became increasingly difficult to manage. The family decided to transition to hospice care, focusing on providing James with comfort and dignity. With the help of hospice professionals, James's pain was well-managed, and he was able to spend his final days at home surrounded by loved ones.

The hospice team provided emotional support to the family, helping them navigate their grief and find peace in knowing they honoured James's wishes.

Examples and Scenarios

Example 2

Supporting the Family

Mark's mother, Helen, had been living with advanced dementia. As her condition progressed, the family struggled with the emotional and physical demands of her care. They decided to seek palliative care to improve Helen's quality of life and support the family. The palliative care team provided symptom management, emotional support, and guidance on Helen's care.

The family found relief in knowing that Helen's needs were being met with compassion and expertise, allowing them to focus on creating meaningful moments together.

Conclusion: Letting Go with Dignity

Hospice and palliative care are not about giving up but about providing the best possible quality of life during the final stages of an illness. These services ensure that your loved one can go with dignity, free from pain, and surrounded by compassion and support. By embracing hospice and palliative care, you are honouring your loved one's wishes and ensuring they receive the respectful and loving care they deserve.

Key Takeaways:
- Hospice Care focuses on comfort and support during the end-of-life stage, addressing physical, emotional, and spiritual needs.
- Palliative Care provides symptom relief and improved quality of life for individuals with serious illnesses at any stage.
- Both approaches prioritize dignity, comfort, and respect for the patient's wishes.
- Hospice and palliative care support families through respite care, bereavement support, and education.
- Embracing these services ensures that your loved one's final journey is peaceful, dignified, and filled with compassion.

By understanding and utilizing hospice and palliative care, you can provide your loved one with the comfort and dignity they deserve, making their final days meaningful and serene.

12.5
What If the Person Outlives You?

Caring for a loved one is a deeply fulfilling yet challenging journey, and one question that may weigh on your mind is, "What if the person I'm caring for outlives me?" While it's a difficult topic to contemplate, it's essential to plan for such scenarios to ensure that your loved one receives the care and support they need even after you're no longer able to provide it. By putting plans in place, you can find peace of mind knowing that your loved one will be in good hands when the time comes.

Assessing the Situation

Understanding Longevity
Consider Lifespan: Evaluate your loved one's current health status, age, and family history to estimate their life expectancy. While it's impossible to predict with certainty, understanding potential longevity can help inform your planning process.

Assess Support Systems: Identify family members, friends, or professionals who may be willing and able to step in and provide care if needed. Assess the availability of community resources, such as social services or support groups, that can offer assistance.

Creating a Care Plan

Documenting Preferences
Discuss Wishes: Have open conversations with your loved one about their preferences for care in the event of your absence. Document their wishes regarding living arrangements, medical treatment, financial management, and other important aspects of their life.

Legal Documentation: Work with an attorney to create legal documents such as a will, power of attorney, and advance directives. Designate a trusted individual as the executor of the estate and power of attorney for healthcare and finances.

Building a Support Network by Engaging Family and Friends

Identify Caregivers: Reach out to family members and friends who may be willing to take on caregiving responsibilities if necessary. Discuss expectations, roles, and responsibilities to ensure everyone is prepared and willing to provide support.

Community Resources: Explore community resources and support services that can assist with caregiving, such as respite care, home health services, or adult day programs. Connect with local agencies or organizations that specialize in supporting older adults or individuals with specific needs.

Securing Financial Stability & Planning

Financial Planning: Review your loved one's financial situation and consider how to ensure their financial stability in your absence. Set up automatic bill payments, organize important financial documents, and designate a trusted individual to manage finances if needed.

Long-Term Care Insurance: Investigate long-term care insurance options that can help cover the costs of care in the event of extended illness or disability. Consult with a financial advisor to explore strategies for maximizing assets and minimizing financial burden.

Communicating Your Plans and being Transparent

Open Communication: Discuss your care plans with your loved one and other family members to ensure everyone is aware of their responsibilities and roles. Encourage open dialogue about potential scenarios and how they will be addressed.

Documentation and Accessibility: Keep important documents, such as wills, advance directives, and contact lists, in a secure yet accessible location. Provide copies to trusted individuals and ensure they understand where to find these documents when needed.

Reviewing and Updating Plans

Regular Assessments: Periodically review and update your care plans to reflect changes in your loved one's health status, personal preferences, or support network. Stay informed about new resources or services that may benefit your loved one's care.

Family Discussions: Schedule regular family meetings to discuss any updates or changes to the care plan and address any concerns or questions that arise. Keep lines of communication open to ensure everyone remains on the same page.

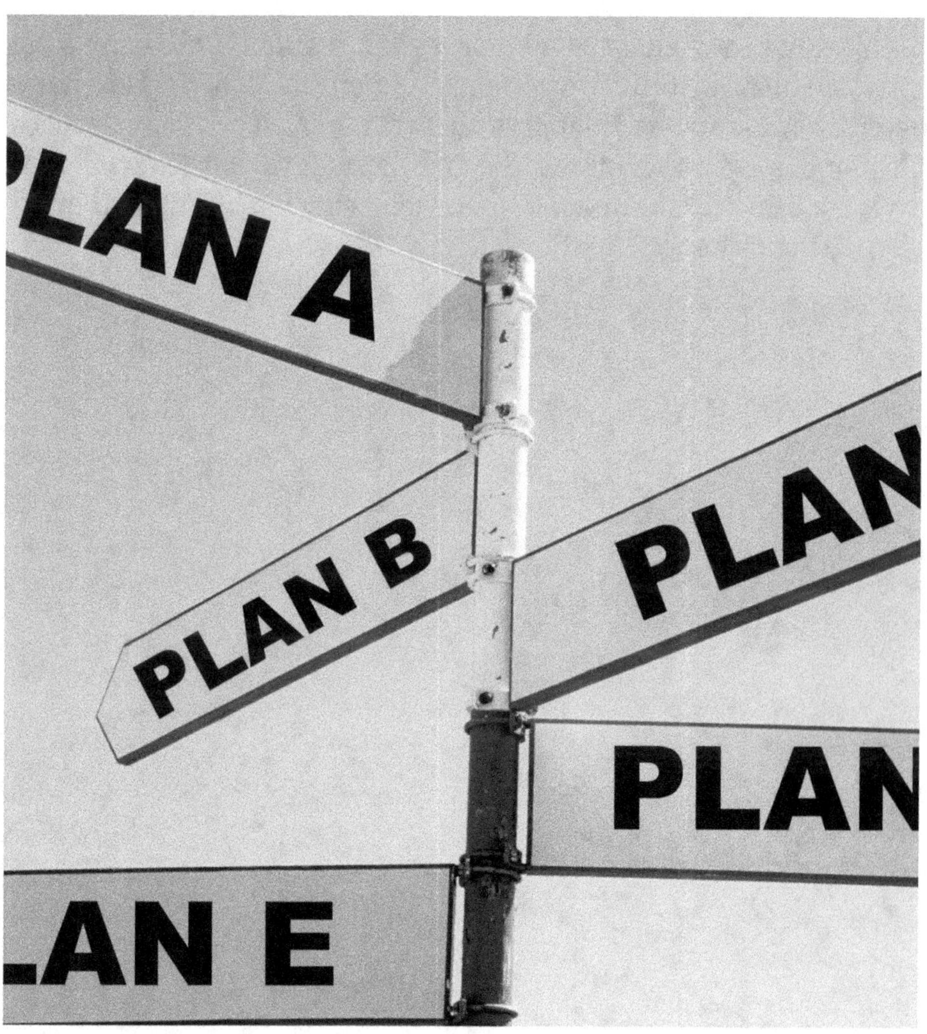

Conclusion: Ensuring Continuity of Care

Planning for the possibility that your loved one may outlive you is an essential aspect of long-term care planning. By assessing the situation, creating a comprehensive care plan, building a support network, securing financial stability, communicating your plans, and regularly reviewing and updating them, you can ensure continuity of care and peace of mind for both yourself and your loved one.

While it may be a challenging topic to address, taking proactive steps now can alleviate future uncertainty and ensure that your loved one receives the care and support they need, even in your absence. Remember, by preparing for the unexpected, you're demonstrating your enduring commitment to their well-being and ensuring they are in good hands for years to come.

Papa's Last Song.

In the symphony of life's grand score,
Each note a memory we adore,
A melody of joy and pain,
Of sunshine bursts and gentle rain.

This journey, like a farewell tour,
We played our parts, we asked for more,
The highs and lows, the sweet refrain,
A dance of laughter, a touch of strain.

The beginning of the end draws near,
But let us face it without fear,
With gratitude for every song,
For every right, for every wrong.

Thank you for a great life's sound,
For harmonies that know no bound,
For every chord, for every rhyme,
n the endless march of time.

Though any day is not to choose,
To bid this world a solemn adieu,
Today I stand, with head held high,
For today is a good day to die.

Yet in this moment, bold and bright,
I feel the warmth of life's pure light,
And know within, we've lived it all,
With hearts that answered every call.

So as the final notes fade low,
And we prepare to let them go,
Remember this, our song so true,
Was beautiful because of you.

In the silence that follows the applause,
In the quiet of life's pause,
Know that we danced, we lived, we tried,
In the harmony where love abides.

For in the end, it's clear to see,
We've made our mark, our symphony,
With dignity, we've said goodbye,
Knowing today's a good day to die.

CONCLUSION

YOU, ME & THE OTHER ONE

"In caregiving, it's not just about you or me; it's about us, together, with the other one. Balancing our needs and theirs is the heart of compassionate care."

YOU, ME AND THE OTHER ONE

Reflecting on our journey together through "You, Me, and THE OTHER ONE," we've explored the multifaceted world of caregiving, delving into the emotional, psychological, and practical challenges that caregivers face daily. As we've discussed, caregiving is a complex and demanding role that intertwines the needs of THE OTHER ONE, the person you are caring for, with the responsibilities that fall upon ME, the caregiver, and the personal impact it has on MYSELF.

Understanding the Emotional Landscape

One of the key themes we've touched upon is the emotional landscape of caregiving. From dealing with stress and trauma to navigating the daily highs and lows, we've highlighted how vital it is to recognize and address these emotional challenges. By understanding the triggers, both fast and slow, we can better manage our responses and maintain our well-being. Just as I found solace and a sanity check in writing music as "Papa Roy," finding personal outlets and coping mechanisms can be crucial for maintaining your mental health.

The Power of Mindfulness and Resilience

Mindfulness, as we discussed, is like crafting a recipe—carefully balancing the ingredients of our thoughts and emotions to create a harmonious state of mind. Resilience is not just about bouncing back from adversity but about thriving amidst challenges. By nurturing our inner strength and embracing the journey with courage and grace, we can foster a positive caregiving environment.

The Impact of Trauma

Trauma, especially when deep-rooted from past incidents, often leads caregivers and care recipients to rely on their emotional brains rather than their thinking brains. This reliance can result in more triggers and increased stress for both THE OTHER ONE and MYSELF. Recognizing these signs and understanding their origins is essential for mitigating their impact. By addressing trauma head-on, we can improve our caregiving approach and enhance the quality of care we provide.

Finding Comfort in Creativity

Be creative and unlock that side of you. It will leave you with a sense of achievement.

Embracing the Journey

Caregiving is a journey filled with both rewarding moments and daunting challenges. It's about finding balance, seeking support, and maintaining hope. The quotes and poems included in this guide are there to uplift and inspire you, providing moments of reflection and motivation. They serve as gentle reminders that you are not alone in this journey.

A Source of Comfort and Guidance

Ultimately, I hope this guide becomes a source of comfort and a practical tool to help you navigate the caregiving journey. The insights and strategies discussed aim to support you in managing the day-to-day responsibilities of caring for THE OTHER ONE, while also taking care of ME and MYSELF. It's about creating a sustainable and compassionate approach to caregiving that honour's the well-being of everyone involved.

Your Daily Routine

Consider your daily routine—how it starts and how it flows. Disruptions in this routine can act as slow triggers, gradually building up stress. By recognizing these triggers and finding ways to mitigate them, you can create a more stable and supportive environment for both yourself and the person you care for.

First Time Carers!

Get your hands dirty as soon as you can. Get used to those tasks that appear unpleasant. Once you get over the initial shock of doing this, you will get used to it. There is support out there. There are coaches and trainers who can show you how to do things, if you need the help.

Looking Ahead

As you move forward, remember to prioritize self-care, seek professional help when needed, and build a support network. Share your experiences, learn from others, and continue to grow in your caregiving role. Each day is an opportunity to make a positive impact, not only on THE OTHER ONE but also on ME and MYSELF.

Thank you for allowing me to be a part of your journey. I hope the stories, insights, and creative expressions shared here bring you strength and solace. Together, we can create a caregiving experience that is both nurturing and fulfilling, where the well-being of all—You, Me, and THE OTHER ONE—is cherished and supported.

APPENDICES

Appendices in a care book are like a superhero's utility belt—packed with extra goodies to save the day! They're the backstage pass to deeper insights, housing tools, checklists, and bonus materials that amplify the book's core wisdom. In the caregiving world, where every day brings new challenges, appendices are the secret weapons that turn knowledge into action. So, while they might lurk at the back, their impact is anything but hidden!

General Resources for Carers

1. Alzheimer's Association: www.alz.org
2. Family Caregiver Alliance: www.caregiver.org
3. Carers Trust: www.carers.org
4. National Alliance for Caregiving: www.caregiving.org

United Kingdom

1. Carers UK: www.carersuk.org
2. NHS Carers Direct: www.nhs.uk/conditions/social-care-and-support-guide/support-and-benefits-for-carers/
3. Age UK: www.ageuk.org.uk
4. The Princess Royal Trust for Carers: www.carers.org
5. Alzheimer's Society (UK): www.alzheimers.org.uk
6. National Autistic Society: www.autism.org.uk
7. MS Society (UK): www.mssociety.org.uk
8. Cerebral Palsy UK: www.cerebralpalsy.org.uk
9. Headway - the brain injury association: www.headway.org.uk

USA

1. AARP Caregiving Resource Center: www.aarp.org/caregiving
2. Eldercare Locator: www.eldercare.acl.gov/Public/Index.aspx
3. Caregiver Action Network: www.caregiveraction.org
4. National Institute on Aging: www.nia.nih.gov/health/caregiving
5. Alzheimer's Association: www.alz.org
6. Autism Society: www.autism-society.org
7. National Multiple Sclerosis Society: www.nationalmssociety.org
8. Cerebral Palsy Foundation: www.yourcpf.org
9. Brain Injury Association of America: www.biausa.org

Canada

1. Canadian Caregiver Coalition: www.ccc-ccan.ca
2. Alzheimer Society of Canada: www.alzheimer.ca/en/help-support/im-caregiver
3. Canadian Virtual Hospice: www.virtualhospice.ca

4. Family Caregivers of British Columbia: www.familycaregiversbc.ca
5. Autism Canada: www.autismcanada.org
6. Multiple Sclerosis Society of Canada: www.mssociety.ca
7. Cerebral Palsy Association in Alberta: www.cpalberta.com
8. Brain Injury Canada: www.braininjurycanada.ca

Australia

1. Carers Australia: www.carersaustralia.com.au
2. Dementia Australia: www.dementia.org.au
3. Australian Government Carer Gateway: www.carergateway.gov.au
4. Carers Victoria: www.carersvictoria.org.au
5. Autism Spectrum Australia (Aspect): www.autismspectrum.org.au
6. MS Australia: www.msaustralia.org.au
7. Cerebral Palsy Alliance: www.cerebralpalsy.org.au
8. Brain Injury Australia: www.braininjuryaustralia.org.au

Mental Health Resources

Global Resources

1. Mental Health Foundation: www.mentalhealth.org.uk
2. Mind: www.mind.org.uk
3. National Institute of Mental Health (NIMH): www.nimh.nih.gov
4. World Health Organization (WHO): www.who.int/mental_health
5. International Association for Suicide Prevention (IASP): www.iasp.info

United Kingdom

1. NHS Mental Health Services: www.nhs.uk/mental-health
2. Samaritans: www.samaritans.org
3. Rethink Mental Illness: www.rethink.org
4. YoungMinds: www.youngminds.org.uk
5. Dementia UK: www.dementiauk.org
6. National Autistic Society: www.autism.org.uk

United States

1. Mental Health America (MHA): www.mhanational.org
2. National Alliance on Mental Illness (NAMI): www.nami.org
3. Substance Abuse and Mental Health Services Administration (SAMHSA): www.samhsa.gov
4. American Foundation for Suicide Prevention (AFSP): www.afsp.org
5. Autism Society: www.autism-society.org
6. Alzheimer's Association: www.alz.org

Canada

1. Canadian Mental Health Association (CMHA): www.cmha.ca
2. Centre for Addiction and Mental Health (CAMH): www.camh.ca
3. Kids Help Phone: www.kidshelpphone.ca
4. Crisis Services Canada: www.crisisservicescanada.ca
5. Autism Canada: www.autismcanada.org
6. Alzheimer Society of Canada: www.alzheimer.ca

Australia

- Beyond Blue: www.beyondblue.org.au
- Lifeline Australia: www.lifeline.org.au
- Headspace: www.headspace.org.au
- Black Dog Institute: www.blackdoginstitute.org.au
- Autism Awareness Australia: www.autismawareness.com.au
- Dementia Australia: www.dementia.org.au

These resources provide a wealth of information, support, and services for those experiencing mental health challenges and for caregivers seeking to improve their caregiving skills while maintaining their

ACKNOWLEDGEMENTS

I extend my heartfelt gratitude to all who have contributed to the creation of "Me, Myself and the OTHER ONE." Firstly, I wish to express my appreciation to the individuals whose stories have inspired this work. Your courage and resilience have illuminated the pages of this book, and I am deeply honored to have had the opportunity to share your experiences.

To the photographers whose captivating images adorn these pages, sourced from copyright-free platforms such as Canvas, thank you for your artistry and generosity. Additionally, I am grateful for the additional photographs captured by myself, Roy Langstaffe, which have enriched the visual narrative of this book.

Furthermore, I wish to acknowledge that any person mentioned in this book has had their names altered to safeguard their privacy and protect their identity.

Lastly, to my family, friends, and colleagues who have provided unwavering support and encouragement throughout this endeavor. Special mention to Angela, Jake, Charlie and Laurie. I am profoundly grateful. Your belief in me has been a constant source of strength, and I am indebted to each of you for your unwavering support.

With deepest appreciation,

Roy Langstaffe

Disclaimer

© 2024 Roy Langstaffe. All rights reserved. No part of this publication, "Me, Myself and THE OTHER ONE," may be reproduced, distributed, or transmitted in any form or by any means, including photocopying, recording, or other electronic or mechanical methods, without the prior written permission of the publisher, except in the case of brief quotations embodied in critical reviews and certain other noncommercial uses permitted by copyright law.

The information contained in this book is for general informational purposes only. The author assumes no responsibility for errors or omissions in the contents of the book. The information is provided on an 'as is' basis with no guarantees of completeness, accuracy, usefulness, or timeliness.

This book is not intended to provide medical, legal, or financial advice. Readers are advised to seek the services of a qualified professional in these fields.

While the author has made every effort to ensure that the information in this book is correct, the author does not assume and hereby disclaims any liability to any party for any loss, damage, or disruption caused by errors or omissions, whether such errors or omissions result from negligence, accident, or any other cause.
This book may contain links to external websites that are not provided or maintained by or in any way affiliated with the author. Please note that the author does not guarantee the accuracy, relevance, timeliness, or completeness of any information on these external websites.

Photos provided by Canva are copyright-free. All other photos are by Roy Langstaffe.

www.ingramcontent.com/pod-product-compliance
Lightning Source LLC
Chambersburg PA
CBHW070823250726
48662CB00003B/1060